"This book provides an easy-to-follow, comprehensive program for losing weight and keeping it off. Unlike many books on this topic, the strategies in this book are based on proven psychological principles. I recommend this workbook to anyone who struggles to lose weight and live a healthier lifestyle."

—Martin M. Antony, Ph.D., ABPP, professor of psychology at Ryerson University in Toronto, ON, Canada, and author of *When Perfect Isn't Good Enough*

"Given the lack of effective tools to assist people in their weight struggles, this book fills an important gap. It provides evidence-based strategies for weight management, addresses problematic thoughts and behaviors, and offers long-term lifestyle solutions for healthy eating, exercise, and maintaining a positive body image. This book is a valuable resource for both consumers struggling with weight issues and the clinicians who help them."

—Traci McFarlane, Ph.D., C.Psych., staff psychologist and clinical team leader at Toronto General Hospital and assistant professor at the University of Toronto

"Changing the way you think is key to losing weight and eating more mindfully. This straightforward, easy-to-read guide helps illuminate the thoughts and behaviors that may be standing in the way. You'll learn essential skills that will take you far on your journey toward a healthier you!"

—Susan Albers, Psy.D., author of *50 Ways to Soothe Yourself Without Food, Eating Mindfully, and Eat, Drink, and Be Mindful*

"This is a fantastic tool for individuals seeking to find an exit ramp from the freeways and cloverleaves of dieting, weight regain, and more dieting. Completing the program laid out in this book will help almost anyone get their life and eating habits back under control, determine a long-term path toward a healthier lifestyle, and develop a more contented acceptance of their own body. It should be a required tool in every weight management clinic on the planet, and I feel strongly that it should be required reading for every family practice physician and health care provider in North America."

—Julie Janeway, author of *The Real Skinny on Weight Loss Surgery* and coauthor of *The Encyclopedia of Obesity*

D0896906

The Cognitive Behavioral Workbook *for* Weight Management

A STEP-BY-STEP PROGRAM

MICHELE LALIBERTE, PH.D.
RANDI E. MCCABE, PH.D.
VALERIE TAYLOR, MD, PH.D.

New Harbinger Publications, Inc.

Publisher's Note

Distributed in Canada by Raincoast Books

Copyright © 2009 by Michele Laliberte, Randi McCabe, and Valerie Taylor
New Harbinger Publications, Inc.
5674 Shattuck Avenue
Oakland, CA 94609
www.newharbinger.com

Cover design by Amy Shoup
Text design by Michele Waters-Kermes
Acquired by Tesilya Hanauer

FSC
Mixed Sources
Product group from well-managed
forests and other controlled sources

Cert no. SW-COC-002283
www.fsc.org
© 1996 Forest Stewardship Council

Printed in the United States of America

Library of Congress Cataloging-in-Publication Data on file with the publisher

11   10   09

10   9   8   7   6   5   4   3   2   1

First printing

This book is dedicated to our patients, who have inspired us with their courage, strength, perseverance, and hope in the face of ongoing struggle.

Contents

Acknowledgments

Preparing this book has been a labor of love that has involved many people along the way. First and foremost, we would like to thank all of the patients we have worked with over the years, who have trusted us with their struggles, taught us about courage and strength, and inspired us to write this book.

We would like to thank the staff at New Harbinger Publications. We are grateful to Catharine Sutker for helping to get this project off the ground. We would also like to thank Tesilya Hanauer, Jess Beebe, and Karen Stein for their encouragement and valuable feedback on the manuscript.

We extend a special thank-you to our colleagues and friends for their helpful input and comments: Anne Williams, Amy Wojtowicz, Jacquelyn MacKenzie, Max Taylor, Annette Taylor, Judy Bartlett, Terri-Ann Tabak, Dr. Yoni Freedhoff, and Julie Janeway. Most important, we would like to thank our families for their support and understanding throughout this process: Neville Jackson, Bryce Jackson, Nicholas Jackson, Russell Jackson, William Harper, Liam Harper-McCabe, and Brendan Harper-McCabe.

Introduction

Take a moment to consider the following questions:

- *Are you tired of struggling with your weight?*

- *Have you tried numerous weight-loss programs without lasting success?*

- *Are you worried about your weight for health reasons but don't know what to do?*

- *Do you struggle with body dissatisfaction?*

- *Do you engage in emotional eating?*

- *Do you wish you could be more physically fit, but hate exercising?*

- *Are you confused about what you should do in your efforts to control your weight?*

If you answered yes to any of these questions, this book will provide you with some answers, strategies, and direction.

Whether you hope to improve your health or want to feel better about your body, this book offers you a weight management plan you can count on. In our work with clients struggling with weight-related issues, and with other health care professionals, we have often wished we had a self-help book we could recommend that addressed weight management, health, and body image in a realistic way. In developing this book, we have attempted to provide information that is based on research wherever possible. The purpose of this book is to help you choose and implement a realistic weight management program that will improve your health, body image, or both. This book will show you how to make systematic changes that can last a lifetime.

HOW TO USE THIS BOOK

This is an action-oriented workbook. It is about learning; self-assessment; exploration of thoughts, feelings, and behaviors; and making behavioral changes. To make these changes, you will need to commit to engaging in the exercises and activities. Of course, just reading this book will heighten your awareness, but if you don't *do* anything, then you will not see any changes. You can follow this book on your own or with the support of a therapist or your medical doctor.

Here are some tips for success on your journey:

- Remember that your focus needs to be on finding a weight management plan that you can live with for the long term—for a *lifetime*.

- Think of this journey as an experiment. We will provide you with a number of weight management options. Your own experiences should guide you. As you go along, you may change your mind about the option that is best for you.

- Try to make changes at a reasonable pace. Small changes that you can sustain will work better in the long run than trying to change everything at once.

- Find time each day to complete the exercises—book it in your calendar or it won't get done. Make yourself a priority in your schedule. You are worth it!

- Engage your support systems to help you make changes. Support from family and friends can make all the difference.

- Reward yourself. It is not easy to break old habits and confront your challenges. You may need to find satisfying rewards that are not related to food.

CHAPTER 1

What You Need to Know About Weight and Weight Loss *Before* You Get Started

You may hope this book will help you to lose weight, or at least help you to prevent weight gain. Before you choose the weight management approach that best suits you, however, you need to have the necessary information to make an informed decision. The aim of this chapter is to bring you up to date on the current scientific understanding of weight, weight loss, and how the body regulates weight.

Weight Management for *Real* People: Meet Five Such People

You have your own story of your weight concerns. Sometimes it's helpful to hear about other people's experiences. We would like you to meet five people who are struggling with their weight: Jim, Karen, Janice, Carlos, and Jennifer. We will use their experiences throughout this book to demonstrate how to implement changes in your own life.

Jim

Weight: 356 lb.
Height: 6'1"
Body Mass Index (BMI): 47

Jim is a fifty-one-year-old shift worker at an auto plant. As a young man, he played football in high school and was known for his physical strength. His job required him to be physically active until around age forty, when he was promoted to a foreman's position. His weight then began to increase rapidly as his work became more sedentary, and he found it difficult to remain active because of his schedule. As his weight climbed to 356 pounds, it became difficult for Jim to walk the floor and supervise the people working for him. His boss expressed concern at his lack of supervision and suggested that it could result in a poor performance review.

Jim's wife works as a nurse's aide. Although she's worried about Jim's weight, their schedules make it difficult for them to have regular meals together with their two daughters. They often rely on convenience foods. When Jim's schedule won't allow him to eat with his family, he typically turns to fast food or a local all-day-breakfast diner. His physician has expressed concern about Jim's weight, especially since he was recently diagnosed with type 2 diabetes and has elevated cholesterol and blood pressure. Jim's doctor recommended that he try to lose weight, so he and his wife joined a commercial weight-loss program. Jim was successful at losing a small amount of weight but, with his schedule, found it very difficult to follow the plan. Jim is worried about his job and his health, and he's frustrated by his inability to get his weight under control. His physician recently suggested he consider bariatric (weight loss) surgery.

Karen

Weight: 236 lb.
Height: 5'4"
BMI: 40.5

Karen is a forty-two-year-old account manager at her local bank. As a child, she was on the larger side and was teased by her peers at school about her weight. Her mother was also critical of her weight and had Karen on various weight-loss programs starting at age ten. In her twenties, Karen successfully lost weight through a commercial weight-loss program. About twice a month, she would "fall off her diet" and eat a large amount of food. These binge episodes were infrequent enough that she didn't worry too much about them. Karen got married and had a son. Shortly afterward, she became depressed and was prescribed medication for her mood. In her thirties, Karen and her husband separated. During the daytime, she struggled to return to the regimented eating of her twenties but began to experience frequent binge episodes in the evening. Her weight steadily climbed. Karen experienced difficulties with back pain and went to her physician for help, but she felt that her doctor attributed it entirely to her weight and didn't properly investigate the complaint. She began to feel uncomfortable going to doctor's appointments and, as a result, hasn't had a physical in years. Karen worries about her health and is desperately unhappy with her appearance.

Janice

Weight: 196 lb.
Height: 5'7"
BMI: 30.7

Janice is a successful thirty-eight-year-old business executive who is married with three children. Her father was a large man, and she and her sister are tall, full-bodied women. Although Janice was never "small," she didn't worry about her weight until after her third child was born. She had gained about twenty pounds with each pregnancy, and her physician suggested that she might want to try a commercial weight-loss program. She found it embarrassing that her physician was concerned enough about her weight to make this suggestion. Shortly afterward, her father had emergency open-heart surgery following a mild heart attack. This event prompted her to take her own health more seriously. Although Janice was motivated to change her lifestyle, her work often required her to travel. She found it difficult to control her portion sizes when eating at restaurants and had trouble sticking to an exercise program when on the road. When they were at home, she and her husband tended to cook healthy meals, but they both loved to snack on potato chips in the evening while watching television. Janice is a disciplined person in most aspects of her life and wants a sensible, realistic approach to weight loss.

Carlos

Weight: 187 lb.
Height: 5'8"
BMI: 28.4

Carlos is a thirty-nine-year-old vice principal at his local high school. He is a married father of two, and his wife works as a social worker at a hospital. Carlos's cholesterol levels are elevated, and ever since he was a young man, he has had high blood pressure, which is now successfully controlled on medication. Most of the men in his family have had trouble with high blood pressure, and his uncle and grandfather both had heart attacks at a relatively young age. Carlos cooks the meals in their home and loves to prepare rich gourmet foods when he can. He also likes to pour himself a drink after work and has another glass or two of wine with dinner. He has never really enjoyed formal exercise and prefers to socialize in the evenings with his family and neighbors. His wife worries about his health and has tried to encourage Carlos to cook leaner meals and become more active. Carlos is good natured about her concerns, but he can't quite stick to any plan. He would like to be healthy, but he doesn't want to give up life's pleasures—especially good food.

■ Jennifer

Weight: 153 lb.
Height: 5'6"
BMI: 24.7

Jennifer is twenty-one years old and in her third year of university. She feels frustrated that she seems to have inherited her mother's fuller body. Her mother is also dissatisfied with her own appearance and is always on some new diet program. Over the years, her mother often invited her daughter to join her on her weight-loss programs. Jennifer tried some of these programs, but she would find herself adopting stricter practices than the program guidelines recommended. Although she did lose weight on occasion, the diet attempt would usually end with a "bang": she would end up binge eating. At that point, she would give up on her diet plan and gradually regain her lost weight. Currently, she feels miserable about her weight and uncertain about her eating. She wants to feel better about her weight and believes she just needs to find the right diet approach.

THE TWO BIG CONCERNS: HEALTH AND BODY IMAGE

The two main reasons why people are unhappy with their weight are concerns about their health and dissatisfaction with their appearance. Let's look at each of these in turn.

Do I Really Need to Worry About My Health If I Am Overweight?

There are a number of health problems associated with carrying extra body fat. The more you weigh, the greater the health risks. Extra weight in the form of body fat is associated with an increase in risk factors for cardiovascular disease, type 2 diabetes, stroke, sleep apnea, and certain types of cancers. Excess body weight also worsens certain chronic diseases, such as high blood pressure (hypertension), osteoarthritis, and joint-skeletal problems. However, not everyone who is overweight has health problems. Chapter 2 will focus on helping you to determine your potential health risks.

WILL WEIGHT LOSS IMPROVE MY HEALTH?

Although you might assume that weight loss improves your health, this is not always true. There are health risks associated with weight loss when the diet is too low in calories (less than 800 kilocalories per day) or nutritionally very imbalanced, or if weight loss occurs too rapidly. Intentional, moderate, and nutritionally balanced weight loss, however, is related to positive health outcomes (Gregg and Williamson 2002). In the short term, moderate weight loss is related to improvement in virtually all the risk factors associated with cardiovascular disease and type 2 diabetes (Orzano and Scott 2004). When changes to diet and activity lead to a reduction in the percentage of body fat (as opposed to a loss of fluids or lean body tissue), the rate of death is lowered (Allison et al. 1999). If your goal is to lower your health risks, you will want a weight-loss approach that will specifically reduce body fat and not just overall weight.

HOW MUCH WEIGHT SHOULD I LOSE TO IMPROVE MY HEALTH?

Experts used to recommend that people aim to get their weight into the "healthy/normal" range. Researchers and medical experts now recommend that people aim for a weight loss of 5 to 10 percent of their excess body weight, far less than most people identify as their weight loss goal (Foster, Wadden, Vogt, and Brewer 1997). This is because we know that even moderate weight loss results in improvement of overall health. In practical terms, this means that a person of 220 pounds would aim to lose somewhere between 11 and 22 pounds, and should expect to see improvement in his risk factors with this decrease in weight. Specifically, research shows improvement in blood pressure, low-density lipoprotein (LDL) or "bad" cholesterol, total cholesterol, triglycerides, insulin levels, and cardiorespiratory fitness levels with even this modest amount of weight loss. This amount of weight loss is also related to better glycemic control among diabetics (Gregg and Williamson 2002).

IS WEIGHT LOSS NECESSARY TO IMPROVE HEALTH?

Experts acknowledge that they cannot say whether the health benefits they find in many weight-loss studies are due to positive changes in lifestyle, such as improved diet and increased physical activity, or to the weight loss that results from these changes. Some intriguing studies suggest that body fat may not be the real issue behind many of the health problems associated with obesity. Rather, the most important factor may be physical fitness: what happens to your body (especially your heart and lungs) as a result of being physically active.

Researchers studied over twenty-five thousand men in the normal weight, overweight, and obese categories and followed them for an average of eight and a half years (Barlow et al. 1995; Lee, Blair, and Jackson 1999). Fit men in each category had substantially lower cardiovascular disease and death rates than did the unfit men. Fit but obese men had lower death rates than unfit lean men did. The reality is, however, that overweight and obese men are far less likely to be physically fit than lean men are. These same researchers found that the percentage of fit men drops dramatically as you move up in the weight categories, with less than 10 percent of men in the lean category being unfit, and more than 90 percent of men in the obese category being unfit. Similar percentages were found in women. This pattern may be due to the fact that people in higher weight categories sometimes have difficulty or discomfort with taking part in physical activity. If health concerns are among your reasons for considering weight management, it's important to look at ways to increase your physical activity and fitness levels.

Key Point: Carrying extra body fat increases your health risks. Changes to your lifestyle that result in a 5 to 10 percent drop in body weight are likely to improve your health risks. Becoming physically fit, even if you remain at a higher weight, is also an effective strategy for improving your health.

Will Weight Loss Help Me Feel Better About My Appearance?

Health concerns are considered by many to be the most "legitimate" reason for worrying about your weight. The majority of people, however, hope weight loss will improve their appearance. This is true even for those people who have health concerns (Wadden et al. 2000). People feel that if they lose weight, they will feel more self-confident, have greater self-esteem, and be treated with greater respect.

WHAT'S THE IMPACT OF WEIGHT LOSS ON BODY SATISFACTION?

Research *does* show that body satisfaction improves as people lose weight. People who lose 5 to 15 percent of their body weight experience significant improvement in their body satisfaction, bringing their satisfaction close to normal levels. It's interesting to note, however, that larger weight losses haven't been associated with greater improvements in body image (Foster, Wadden, and Vogt 1997). A person of 220 pounds who loses between 11 and 33 pounds can expect to experience a significant improvement in body satisfaction. Any further weight loss is unlikely to result in greater body satisfaction. This is reassuring, since the weight loss recommended for improved health is within the same range as that likely to result in increased body satisfaction.

I NEED TO LOSE WEIGHT TO FEEL BETTER ABOUT MY BODY, RIGHT?

Actually, you do not need to lose weight to feel better about your body. In fact, weight loss may *not* be a good strategy for improving body image, because most people will inevitably regain the weight they lose, and it's common for people to have a significant drop in body satisfaction when they gain back even a minimal amount of weight. In contrast, research has shown that people experience significant and lasting improvement in body image after taking part in cognitive behavioral therapy (CBT) for body image (Rosen and Cash 1995). Later in this book, we will introduce you to CBT techniques, including two chapters that focus on body image.

> **Key Point:** Losing a relatively small amount of weight (5 to 15 percent) improves body satisfaction, and there is little improvement in body image from further weight loss. You can achieve similar levels of body satisfaction through the use of CBT techniques described later in this book, and this improvement in body satisfaction is more likely to last over time.

UNDERSTANDING BODY WEIGHT

You may have wondered why you struggle with your weight when others around you appear to have little difficulty maintaining their slim figures even when their lifestyles are less than perfect. You may also have wondered why it's so hard to get your body to cooperate. Even if you have successfully lost weight before, it may have been difficult to maintain that weight loss. If you are like many people, you have felt like a failure when you regained the weight you worked so hard to lose. What you read next may surprise you. It may also help you make sense of your own experience.

Why Has Weight Been Such a Struggle for Me?

Most people in Western culture assume that body weight is completely under their personal control. If you are unhappy with your weight, we are told, you simply need to find a good weight loss diet and adhere to it. Once you have lost the weight you wanted to lose, you simply need to adopt a healthy combination of eating and activity, and you will maintain that desired weight, right? In reality, this has proven to be much more difficult to achieve than anyone anticipated.

Genetics or Lifestyle: What Really Determines Weight?

Trying to understand weight control has long been an important research area. One particular area of interest has been the attempt to understand whether a person's weight is due to genetic influences (in other words, what you inherit from your parents) or the environment. To sort this out, scientists looked at identical twins (twins who share the same genetic structure) adopted by different families and raised in different environments (Stunkard et al. 1990). Despite being raised sometimes in very different environments, most of the twins were within five pounds of one another's weight. Stunkard and his colleagues concluded that about 70 percent of the reason for people's weight is their genetics. In other words, biology plays a large role in determining weight.

HOW DO GENETICS PLAY A ROLE IN A PERSON'S WEIGHT?

Our genetic makeup determines not only the basic size we are meant to be, or our "natural body weight," but also how our weight is affected by the lifestyle we lead. We all know people who seem to gain weight by merely looking at food, and others who seem to be able to eat huge quantities with relatively little impact on their weight. Research has confirmed these differences and shown that a person's genetics determine how easily she gains weight in response to overeating. To understand the role of genetics, researchers studied pairs of identical twin men who were overfed one thousand calories per day (Bouchard et al 1990). The researchers found that each twin gained weight at a very similar rate to his *own* twin. In other words, having identical genes resulted in twins gaining weight at the same rate. However, there were big differences in how fast the different pairs of twins gained weight and how much weight they gained. In other words, because each twin pair had genetics that were different from those of the other twin pairs, they gained different amounts of weight at different rates. We would all go up in weight if we were overfed, but our individual genetics would determine how quickly and how much weight we gained. Some people, therefore, are clearly more at risk for weight gain than others. An "unhealthy" lifestyle will quickly lead to weight gain in people at higher genetic risk for obesity and will lead to slower weight gain in people at a lower genetic risk.

SO WHAT ABOUT THE ROLE OF ENVIRONMENT?

The environment, and the lifestyle it encourages, is extremely important in determining whether people become overweight. There is no question that the developed world has created an environment often described as "toxic" (Horgen and Brownell 2002). We have developed foods sweeter, saltier, and richer than ever in human history. These foods are so "convenient" that we have to put little or no physical effort into obtaining and preparing them. We also live in an environment where little physical effort is required for us to complete tasks of daily living. Activity is no longer built into our lifestyle. Both play and work often involve a significant amount of time sitting in front of a screen (a television or computer, for example) and few of us need to move much to get through a typical day. Although this may be pleasurable or "convenient," our bodies were not built for such a small amount of activity. Our bodies are meant to survive on lean foods, and we are meant to be active. You may be genetically at risk for being overweight, but lifestyle causes you to express that risk.

Key Point: Genetics play a very big part in determining our "natural" weight, how quickly we gain, and how much weight we gain in response to an unhealthy lifestyle. Unfortunately, the environment and lifestyle that are common in most developed societies promote overeating and inactivity.

How Can the Body Regulate Weight?

You may find it difficult at first to believe that the body regulates weight, but it's true. In fact, the body is excellent at regulating weight and has been compared to a thermostat that regulates the temperature of a home. As the temperature drops, the thermostat causes the heat to come on. As the temperature rises, the thermostat turns on the air conditioning, thereby ensuring that the household temperature remains within a small range. In a similar manner, when you maintain a consistent lifestyle, your body actively defends your weight. Your weight will naturally fluctuate within a five-to-seven-pound range over the course of the day and will stay within this range over time; the range gradually moves upward as you age. As part of your body's weight regulation system, occasional overeating may lead to a temporary drop in appetite. Similarly, occasional undereating may lead to a temporary increase in appetite.

Scientists are still working very hard to understand all the systems involved in the body's regulation of weight. Although we do not know exactly how the body regulates weight, we do know that it involves a number of complex, interacting mechanisms. Here are some of the key components involved in weight regulation:

- Skeletal muscle metabolism

- Body fat and hormones related to body fat

- The brain (particularly the hypothalamus) and a large number of neurochemicals, which control appetite

- The stomach, which senses the presence of food and sends messages to your brain to tell you when to stop eating

All these systems help the body "defend" your weight.

BUT I'M OVERWEIGHT. HOW CAN MY BODY BE DEFENDING THIS WEIGHT?

We know that the body is good at protecting against short-term overeating. In other words, if you overeat a couple of times a week, your body will easily return you to your usual weight, especially if you have good eating habits and are moderately active. When a person consistently overeats for a sustained period, however, body weight will increase. The person's genetics will determine how quickly the weight gain will occur. We also know from animal studies that when rats are overfed and maintain a high weight for a longer period, their bodies begin to defend that higher weight (Corbett, Stern, and Keesey 1986). In other words, if you maintain a higher weight for long enough (in rats, it's as short as six months), your body may defend this higher weight.

Key Point: The body has many systems that work to help you maintain a stable weight, particularly when you have healthy eating habits and are moderately active. If you gain weight and maintain that higher weight, your body will eventually "defend" that higher weight, even if that weight is associated with health risks.

UNDERSTANDING WEIGHT LOSS

Now that you know the body regulates weight, you may wonder what the secret to weight loss will be. There are so many diet books and programs to choose from that the information and misinformation can seem overwhelming. You may know someone who has successfully lost weight or at least have heard of someone who has successfully lost weight. How did they do it? In this section, we will tell you what is known about weight loss, weight-loss approaches, and people who successfully lose weight. In chapters 2 and 3 we will help you evaluate your own weight management needs and choose the weight management approach that's right for you.

So, Can I Lose Weight and Keep the Weight Off?

The research on the success of weight-loss diets is very clear: people can lose weight. Really, to lose weight, you only need to take in fewer calories than your body needs for maintaining your current weight. The "state-of-the-art" diet programs (those staffed by physicians, dietitians, psychologists, and other health care professionals) show an average weight loss of 7 to 10 percent, with the majority of people unable to lose more than 10 to 15 percent of their body weight (Foster 2006; Jeffrey et al. 2000). Typically, after six months, weight loss slows and plateaus. Due to adaptations within the body, weight loss beyond this point is very difficult to achieve. Although some very low calorie diets (which are often nutritionally and medically risky) result in greater weight loss, rapid weight loss is typically followed by rapid weight gain. When researchers compared the very low calorie groups to the more moderate weight-loss groups at one year, both groups showed similar weight loss, suggesting that the very low calorie group had quickly regained much of the weight they initially lost (Wadden and Berkowitz 2002).

If you follow weight-loss participants over the long term, the majority of these participants regain a third of the lost weight in one year, and most show a gradual return to their original weight within five years (Wilson and Brownell 2000). This occurs regardless of the weight-loss strategy used, and the same result has been found in many different studies. Clearly, if you hope for weight loss, your body's biology—specifically, your body's ability to resist and recover from weight loss—is a force to be reckoned with. To be successful at managing your weight, you will need a plan that takes your body's biology into account. So keep reading!

But I've Heard About This Great New Diet Program!

You may have heard about some new best-selling diet book, or a diet endorsed by a physician, movie star, or psychologist. Such authors may even use what sounds like scientific research to support their claims. The reality is that, as long as a diet reduces your calorie intake, you may in fact lose weight. The problem is in maintaining that weight loss. For all the various diets that have been researched, the results are the same: after weight loss comes a gradual return to the starting weight for the majority of people.

BUT I KNOW SOMEONE WHO SUCCESSFULLY LOST WEIGHT AND KEPT IT OFF!

Everyone seems to know at least one person who has successfully lost weight and maintained that weight loss. Weight-loss scientists, aware of the stories of these "successful weight losers," set out to study these people. In 1994, the National Weight Control Registry was set up. The registry is currently following over five thousand people who have lost a minimum of thirty pounds and maintained that weight loss for a minimum of one year. In fact, the average person on the Weight Control Registry has done even better—losing an average of sixty-six pounds and maintaining this lower weight for an average of five and a half years.

The next step was to study these people in order to better understand their success (McGuire et al. 1999; Wing and Hill 2001). Of the people on the registry, 80 percent are women, with an average age of forty-five years. The average age of men on the registry is forty-nine years. Their average food intake totals 1,380 calories, suggesting they are eating considerably less than the typical 2,000 calories per day for women and 2,400 calories per day for men. The majority have a balanced food intake, with 24 percent of calories from fat, 19 percent from protein, and 56 percent from carbohydrates; this breakdown is consistent with recommendations from food guides around the world. Participants in this study who are on low-carbohydrate diets (recently so popular) maintain their weight loss for less time and are less physically active.

So they are eating less, but what kind of physical activity do successful weight losers do? Over 90 percent of people on the registry report using physical activity to lose weight and to maintain weight loss.

They report exercising about one hour per day, which is the equivalent of walking four miles (7.2 kilometers) per day. In fact, the majority (about 76 percent) walk as a means of physical activity.

Just under half of the successful weight losers report weighing themselves daily, with about a third weighing themselves at least weekly.

In summary, these successful weight losers report maintaining a low-calorie, low-fat diet; high levels of daily physical activity; and regular and frequent monitoring of their weight. This is not the "maintenance" program envisioned by most people who embark on a weight-loss diet. Most people assume that once the diet ends, they will be able to resume "normal" eating and ease up on their physical activity. No doubt this helps to explain why so few people are able to maintain their weight loss over the long term.

Looking at the findings from the study of successful weight losers, you can see what you are up against if you plan on weight loss. As discouraging as the information on weight loss may seem, we believe that, to be successful, you need to know the obstacles that are in front of you. Clearly, one of the obstacles to successful long-term weight loss is your own body, which will persistently try to bring you back to what it feels is your "natural" weight (even if that weight is now a high weight).

For this reason, to have an effective weight management strategy, you need to understand and plan for how the body works. Most commercial diet programs won't include information about the research on weight loss because it might discourage you from buying their products. Our goal is to *truly* inform you and help you to develop a realistic weight management plan that will actually work for you for the rest of your life.

> **Key Point:** As long as a weight-loss approach reduces your calorie intake, you will lose weight. Regardless of the weight-loss approach, however, people seem to gradually and almost inevitably regain the weight they lost within five years. Successful weight losers maintain their weight loss by adhering to a low-calorie diet and engaging in high levels of daily physical activity.

It might seem like a difficult task, but there is good news: you can be healthier and feel good in your body. Keep reading.

SO WHAT *IS* THE GOOD NEWS? HOW DO I MANAGE MY WEIGHT?

After reading the preceding information on weight loss, you may wish you hadn't read this chapter. You may feel angry or discouraged. Or maybe you feel relieved: finally someone has helped you to understand why it has been so hard, perhaps impossible, to lose weight and maintain that weight loss.

Rest assured that we *are* going to offer you a number of weight management options. We simply want to offer you weight management options that you can count on, not just another fad diet that might help you lose weight initially but leaves you feeling like a failure when the weight returns.

The Good News: Realistic Weight Management Options for Health Concerns

There *is* good news. It *is* possible to significantly improve your health using realistic weight management approaches. The first piece of good news is that changing your lifestyle to include a healthy, balanced diet and regular physical activity can significantly reduce your health risks—whether or not you lose weight as a result. Working to increase your physical fitness will be an important component of this approach. We will provide you with a specific plan for optimizing your health if this is the approach that appeals to you.

The second piece of good news is that the amount of weight you would need to lose in order to see significant improvements in your health is quite modest. As you read earlier, a weight loss of only 5 to 10 percent of your body weight is all that's required, or even recommended, to lead to important changes in your health. As you now know, maintaining even this amount of weight loss can be challenging, because your body will likely work to return you to your starting weight. You still have options, however.

The first option is to set up the best possible long-term plan, in line with what we have learned from successful weight losers. This book will help you plan both your eating and activity.

Another alternative is to use medications to help you maintain the lifestyle necessary for sustained weight loss. This book will provide you information on medication options, which you can discuss with your physician.

If your health is greatly compromised because of extreme obesity or you are experiencing significant health problems associated with your weight, you may want to consider surgery as an option. We highly recommend that people who are investigating surgery still make an attempt to follow the healthy lifestyle plan (described in chapter 3). People we have worked with to normalize eating prior to surgery consistently express the view that they felt better prepared for life after surgery because of their more balanced, structured eating.

Weight management, whether it involves adopting a healthy lifestyle or losing weight, is an essential part of taking care of your health. In addition to weight management, however, we recommend that you follow your doctor's advice regarding treatment for any medical symptoms you may be experiencing.

More Good News: Realistic Weight Management Options for Feeling Good About Your Body

There's good news about body image as well—really good news. First, experts feel that weight loss is *not* a recommended strategy for improving body satisfaction. Weight loss may make you feel better about your body at first, but body satisfaction appears to be very sensitive to any weight regain, even small amounts. There are more reliable approaches to feeling good in your body, and we take you through these approaches in our body image chapters. If you are skeptical, feel free to jump ahead and read about improving body image. That being said, feeling good about your eating and activity is, for most people, a necessary starting point to improve body satisfaction. Even if you decide to work on your body image without trying to lose weight, we would still recommend starting with a healthy lifestyle eating and activity plan.

Second, even a modest amount of weight loss (5 to 15 percent of your starting weight) is all that's necessary to have significant improvement in body satisfaction, and more weight loss doesn't seem to make people feel any happier. If you choose to work on losing weight, we still recommend that you complete the chapters on body image, since you may experience some weight regain over time. As described in the previous section on improving your health, you may wish to consider medications that will support your weight loss if you have also been experiencing health problems related to your weight. Weight loss and medication options are discussed in chapter 3.

Finally, surgery is not recommended for issues of body image. It is only recommended for health reasons. However, there's no question that body image is affected positively by the weight loss that results from surgery. Even with surgery, however, some weight regain is expected after the first year or two. We still recommend that you do the work outlined in the chapters on body image.

You now have the scoop on how the body works. It's important to understand this in order to create a realistic plan. Each of the options we will present to you in chapter 3 is based on what we know about how the body regulates weight.

However, for weight management to be successful, you will also have to give serious thought to what *you* can realistically live with. We will take you through a detailed description of each of the weight management options described in chapter 3 and help you evaluate the pros and cons of each approach. Once you make your choice, we will help you to develop a plan that will work for you. We will then guide you in implementing your plan, helping you identify any obstacles and teaching you skills for overcoming these obstacles.

Key Point: It is possible to improve your health and feel better about your body. You can choose to follow a healthy living plan or a weight-loss plan and work on improving your health and body image with either approach. If you choose weight loss, you may want to consider medications that support weight loss. If you are very obese or have significant health problems related to weight, you may want to consider surgery.

CHAPTER 2

Setting Your Goals

Before you decide on the plan that you will follow, you need to clearly identify your goals so that you know what you are working toward. We will encourage you to set goals to work on your personal happiness in addition to your weight management strategy, and not wait for happiness to magically fall in your lap because you lost weight.

A PERSONAL CHECKUP: YOUR WEIGHT AND YOUR HEALTH

Two measures have been used to determine your health risk related to weight: body mass index (BMI) and waist circumference.

Body Mass Index

The BMI is a number based on a person's weight relative to his height. You may have seen a BMI chart in your doctor's office that indicates whether you fall in the "underweight," "normal," "overweight," or "obese" weight range. For most people, as BMI increases into the overweight level and beyond, the risk of weight-related health problems also increases.

To find your weight category, use the table on the following page:

Your Height	Normal Weight BMI: 19–25	Overweight BMI: 26–29	Obese BMI: 30–39	Extremely Obese BMI: 40+
5'0"	97–128 lb.	133–148 lb.	153–199 lb.	204 lb. +
5'1"	100–132 lb.	137–153 lb.	158–206 lb.	211 lb. +
5'2"	104–136 lb.	142–158 lb.	164–213 lb.	218 lb. +
5'3"	107–141 lb.	146–163 lb.	169–220 lb.	225 lb. +
5'4"	110–145 lb.	151–169 lb.	174–227 lb.	232 lb. +
5'5"	114–150 lb.	156–174 lb.	180–234 lb.	240 lb. +
5'6"	118–155 lb.	161–179 lb.	186–241 lb.	247 lb. +
5'7"	121–159 lb.	166–185 lb.	191–249 lb.	256 lb. +
5'8"	126–164 lb.	171–190 lb.	197–256 lb.	262 lb. +
5'9"	128–169 lb.	176–195 lb.	203–263 lb.	270 lb. +
5'10"	132–174 lb.	181–202 lb.	209–271 lb.	278 lb. +
5'11"	136–179 lb.	186–208 lb.	216–279 lb.	286 lb. +
6'0"	140–184 lb.	191–213 lb.	221–287 lb.	294 lb. +
6'1"	144–189 lb.	197–219 lb.	227–295 lb.	302 lb. +
6'2"	148–194 lb.	202–225 lb.	233–303 lb.	311 lb. +
6'3"	152–200 lb.	208–232 lb.	240–311 lb.	319 lb. +
6'4"	156–205 lb.	213–238 lb.	246–320 lb.	328 lb. +

Or, if you wish to calculate your BMI more precisely, use the formula in the box below:

$$BMI = \frac{\text{weight in kilograms}}{(\text{height in meters})^2} \quad OR \quad \frac{\text{weight in pounds} \times 703}{(\text{height in inches})^2}$$

For example, Carlos is 5 feet 8 inches tall and weighs 187 pounds. This means his BMI is calculated as follows:

$$\frac{187 \times 703}{(68)^2} = \frac{131,461}{4,624} = 28.4$$

Jim (6'1", 298 pounds) and Karen (5'4", 236 pounds) fall in the "extremely" obese range, as their BMIs are above 40. This range is strongly associated with health problems. Janice's weight (5'7", 196 pounds) is in the obese range, which starts at a BMI of 30. Carlos's weight (5'8", 187 pounds) is in the overweight range, falling between a BMI of 25 and 30. Jennifer is dissatisfied with her weight (5'6", 153 pounds), but her BMI of 24.7 is in the "normal" range.

What weight category do you fall in? _____

If you have calculated it, what is your BMI? _____

Waist Circumference

Falling in the overweight or obese range does not guarantee that you will experience diseases related to excess body fat. Your degree of health risk is also related to where you accumulate body fat (Yusuf et al. 2005). If you tend to be "apple" shaped, with most of your body fat in your abdominal area, your health risks are often higher than for people who are "pear" shaped, with most of their body fat in the buttocks, hips, and thighs. The waist circumference (WC) is measured as shown in figure 1.

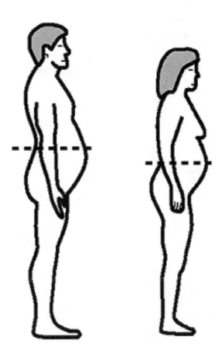

Figure 1. Where to measure your waist circumference

The World Health Organization has suggested the following waist measurement guide for determining risk associated with abdominal obesity (World Health Organization 1998):

	Waist Measurements (just above the hip bones)	
Health Risk Level	Men	Women
Increased Risk	Over 37 in. (94 cm.)	Over 31.5 in. (80 cm.)
Substantially Increased Risk	Over 40 in. (102 cm.)	Over 34.5 in. (88 cm.)

Like many men, Jim and Carlos are both "apple shaped." Even though Carlos falls in the overweight range, his waist measures 38 inches. This may explain some of the medical problems he is already experiencing. Both Karen and Janice are "pear shaped," with waist measurements of 34.5 inches and 32 inches, respectively; their larger waist measurements may mean increased risk of health problems. Jennifer is also "pear shaped," but her waist measurements do not suggest an increased risk of health problems.

What is your waist measurement? _____ (inches/centimeters)

Place a check mark in the appropriate box below if you are at

☐ Increased Risk or ☐ Substantially Increased Risk

What to Do If You Are at Increased Risk

If your BMI or WC fall in a higher-risk range, you may be more likely to experience weight-related health problems. The first step in determining your health goals for weight management is to see your doctor for an assessment of your health risks related to your weight. Research has shown that people who are overweight often avoid going to the doctor for a regular checkup (Fontaine et al. 1998). It can be frightening to hear that you have health risks, but remember that reducing these risks can be your goal for making lifestyle changes. Take the following checklist with you to your doctor. Ask your doctor if lifestyle changes are recommended. Your doctor may also discuss other options for reducing your health risks, such as medications. You should note these on your checklist as well.

Health Risks of Obesity: Medical Assessment Checklist

Take this checklist to your doctor. Record any lifestyle changes or other interventions that your doctor recommends

HEALTH CHECKLIST Check the box ☑ if your doctor indicates this is a health risk for you.	Lifestyle Changes Recommended by Your Doctor	Other Interventions Recommended by Your Doctor
☐ Blood pressure		
Lipid profile:	Lipid profile:	Lipid profile:
☐ Cholesterol		
☐ Triglycerides		
☐ HDL/LDL cholesterol		
☐ Fasting blood sugar		
☐ Sleep apnea		
☐ Nutritional deficiencies: B12, Folate, Ca2+, Mg2+		
☐ Thyroid status		
☐ Depression		
☐ Anxiety		
☐ Binge-eating disorder		
Females: ☐ Gynecological exam ☐ Screen: Polycystic ovarian disease		
Males: ☐ Prostate exam ☐ Screen: Colon cancer		

SETTING YOUR GOALS TO IMPROVE HEALTH

Let's get down to the specifics. What can you do to reduce the health risks associated with being over-weight? In chapter 3, you will consider different weight management approaches, which are intended to improve your health. However, there are specific lifestyle recommendations for decreasing risk factors related to heart disease, diabetes, and certain types of cancer. You may wish to incorporate these strategies in your weight management approach.

Recommended Lifestyle Changes for Good Health

Research has found that certain eating and activity habits are related to good health outcomes. On the left side of the table that follows are lifestyle recommendations, some of which are explained in more detail later. The column on the right indicates the health concerns related to the recommendations; for example, a diet high in soluble fiber is beneficial for a person with heart disease or diabetes.

Lifestyle Recommendation	Target
Diet high in soluble fiber	Heart disease Diabetes
Diet high in insoluble fiber	Diabetes
Minimum of 5 servings of fruits and vegetables; 7 to 8 are even better!	Heart disease Cancer
One dark green and one orange vegetable per day. Citrus fruits and berries are also recommended.	Cancer
Minimum of 2 servings of oily fish per week	Heart disease
Minimum of 2 servings of dairy per day	Heart disease
Diet low in saturated fats	Heart disease
Eating at regular 2- to 4-hour intervals throughout the day	Diabetes
Regular physical activity: 60 minutes built into your daily lifestyle or 150 minutes per week (30 minutes, 5 days per week)	Cancer Heart disease Diabetes

PUTTING THE LIFESTYLE RECOMMENDATIONS INTO PRACTICE

If you are unsure of how to implement the previous recommendations, consider trying some of the following strategies:

Soluble Fiber: Each day, choose one or two foods that are high in soluble fiber, such as oats, legumes (peas, kidney beans, and lentils), brown rice, barley, fruits, some green vegetables (such as broccoli), and potatoes. Alternatively, you may choose a cereal high in soluble fiber (cereals that advertise psyllium, such as bran cereal, are good choices).

Insoluble Fiber: Examples of foods high in insoluble fiber include wheat bran, whole grains, skin of fruits and vegetables, and seeds. Aim to include sources of insoluble fiber in your daily meal plan.

Fruits and Vegetables: *Always* include a fruit or vegetable in every meal or snack, and you will meet your goal. Have berries or citrus for breakfast, carrots for lunch, and a dark green vegetable for dinner.

Oily Fish: Choose an oily fish (like salmon, trout, or sardines) and have that fish once a week for dinner and once for lunch or a snack, perhaps in a sandwich or on crackers.

Dairy: You need to have at least two servings of dairy foods per day. If your breakfast and all snacks include a dairy choice (milk, yogurt, cottage cheese, or cheese), you will get there.

A Diet Low in Saturated Fats: Choose a meatless lunch a few times a week; instead of eating meat, get your protein from peanut butter, hummus, a bean salad, or baked beans. Another simple way to lower your intake of saturated fat is to cook with vegetable oils and use margarine without hydrogenated fats in place of lard or butter.

Physical Activity: Chapter 6 will help you plan physical activity to suit your needs.

Let's Get Specific: Your Food and Activity Goals

We suggest that you start with no more than three food goals. Below, see what Janice chose as her goals; Janice's father had a heart attack, so she's most concerned about her heart health.

■ Janice's Goals

Food Goal 1: *I'm going to add a serving of bran cereal high in psyllium to my usual cereal in the morning.*

Food Goal 2: *I will have a banana and berries on my cereal in the morning, baby carrots and a piece of fruit with my lunch, and at least a cup of cooked veggies with supper.*

Food Goal 3: *I already cook with vegetable oil, but I will buy margarine without hydrogenated fats instead of butter.*

Activity Goal: *I will plan my activity in chapter 6, but I'm thinking of walking—they almost always have treadmills in the hotels I travel to.*

YOUR GOALS

The health concern I want to focus on: _____

Food Goal 1: _____

Food Goal 2: _____

Food Goal 3: _____

Activity Goal: _____

Take the food goals you have set here and work them into the detailed eating plan you will develop in chapter 5.

Measuring Health Changes Over Time

If you decide to make the recommended changes to your lifestyle, you may also wish to measure any reduction of your risk factors. For example, you can monitor your risk factors for heart disease and diabetes over time through blood work ordered by your doctor. Use the following tables to track your progress. You can record the target range you are aiming for based on your doctor's recommendations.

HEART DISEASE: RISK FACTORS

In the case of heart disease, the risk factors most commonly measured are blood pressure, low-density lipoprotein (LDL) "bad" cholesterol, total cholesterol, and triglycerides.

Risk Factors	Starting Measures	Six-Month Follow-Up	Target Range
Blood Pressure			
LDL Cholesterol			
Total Cholesterol			
Triglycerides			

TYPE 2 DIABETES: RISK FACTORS

Risk factors for type 2 diabetes that should be measured include sugar control and risk (hemoglobin AIC) and fasting sugars.

Risk Factors	Starting Measures	Six-Month Follow-Up	Target Range
Hemoglobin AIC			
Fasting Sugars			

If You Plan to Lose Weight: Setting a Realistic Goal

If your weight management strategy involves weight loss (see chapter 3), you will need to set a realistic goal. As you learned in chapter 1, in order to benefit your health, you only need to lose 5 to 10 percent of your excess body weight. What does that mean for you? Calculate your weight loss goal below.

Examples:

Carlos's weight-loss goal range:
= (187 lb. x .05) − (187 lb. x .10) = 9.35 lb to 18.7 lb

Karen's weight-loss goal range:
= (236 lb. x .05) − (236 lb. x .10) = 11.8 lb to 23.6 lb

Your weight-loss goal range = Current weight x .05 − current weight x .10

= _____ x .05 − _____ x .10

= _____ − _____

WHAT IMPACT DOES YOUR WEIGHT HAVE ON YOUR QUALITY OF LIFE?

Your weight may be affecting the quality of your life because of the limitations it places on your mobility. Far more common, however, are the limitations that people place on themselves because of their weight. If you are dissatisfied with or embarrassed by your body, you may avoid certain activities. If this is true for you, we strongly encourage you to work through the body image chapters in this workbook. Let's look at the ways in which concerns about weight could be limiting your quality of life.

Self-Worth

Most critical to your overall happiness is your self-worth, or how you feel about yourself as a person. Dieters are particularly vulnerable to low self-worth, as repeated diet failures may contribute to decreased self-esteem (Stotland and Zuroff 1990).

Jennifer feels that she is less worthwhile as a person when her weight is above where she wants it to be. This leads her to feel insecure and uncomfortable in social situations.

Family Life

Your size or concerns about your body and appearance can affect your family activities and relationships.

Jim didn't feel that he could help coach his daughter's soccer team, because just walking made him tired. He also felt embarrassed about his size, since he used to pride himself on being an athlete.

Romantic Relationships

Your body size and body image concerns can affect either the quality of your current relationship, if you have one, or your ability and willingness to enter into a romantic relationship.

Karen would like to be in a relationship, but she feels so unattractive that she doesn't even attempt to meet people and can't stand the thought of someone touching her or holding her. Her discomfort with physical intimacy contributed to her marital difficulties. When they were still together, Karen's husband told her that he loved her just the way she was, but she would purposefully go to bed later than he did to avoid physical contact.

Work and School Life

Your body size may have a direct impact on your ability to engage in certain jobs and perform at work.

Despite direct feedback from his boss, Jim finds it challenging to keep up with the physical demands of his job.

Your body image concerns can also affect your work life in more indirect ways by affecting your mood, concentration, motivation, and interest.

Jennifer is so preoccupied with her weight that she has difficulty focusing on her school studies.

Leisure Activities

You may find that your size or your body image concerns interfere with your willingness to participate in enjoyable activities.

Karen's back problems make it difficult for her to return to the physical or pleasurable activities she once enjoyed. She can't imagine going to a gym or spa, because she feels too self-conscious about her size.

Social Life

Your weight and feelings about your body size and appearance may interfere with your interest and enjoyment in social activities and friendships.

Jennifer has withdrawn from her friends and no longer goes out due to her body image concerns.

Finances

Your weight issues may also have an impact on your wallet. You may frequently eat out because of your busy schedule, leading to weight gain and increased food expenses. You may have to buy new clothes frequently because your weight fluctuates with your dieting patterns. You may pay high fees for commercial diet programs. You may also have additional health care costs related to your weight. For example, you may require physical therapy for weight-related pain and joint problems, leaving you with less money for other priorities and pleasures.

Karen has ongoing costs for chiropractic and physical therapy treatments for her back pain.

Use the worksheet provided to help you examine the impact of weight on your life.

Impact of Weight Worksheet

For each life area below, consider the impact of your weight and body image concerns. You may feel that only a few boxes apply to you; if so, that's okay.

Life Area	How does your weight physically limit you in this area?	How do body image concerns affect this area of your life?	How would this be different if your weight changed?
Self-Worth			
Family Life			
Romantic Relationships			
Work Life			
Leisure Activities			
Social Life			
Finances			

Worksheet Review

Now that you have completed the Impact of Weight Worksheet, let's step back and examine the effect that weight has had on your quality of life. Answer the questions below in the space provided.

What life areas are affected by your actual physical size?

_____

_____

What life areas are affected by your body image or appearance concerns?

_____

_____

Choose three things that you value and are putting off because of physical limitations or body image concerns:

1. _____

2. _____

3. _____

Give some thought to why you are waiting to start living your life. If it's because your size limits you physically, ask yourself if you are *sure* there is no way around these limitations. Do you really have to wait until you lose weight? If you are waiting because you feel embarrassed about your weight, then working on body image should be a real priority for you. Doing the things on this list can become part of your goals as you address your body image concerns in chapters 10 and 11.

Karen thought she needed to be at a certain weight in order to be happy with herself. She tried many weight-loss programs to achieve this goal. Each weight-loss success eventually ended in failure as she regained what she had lost, plus more. Karen found that over the years she felt worse and worse about herself. Her discomfort with her body led her to avoid physical intimacy with her husband, which contributed to emotional distance in her marriage and its eventual breakup. Her physical health has deteriorated, as she avoids going to her doctor because of her doctor's focus on her weight. She is pretty sure that her physical risks have increased but has avoided thinking about it and hasn't had a routine physical examination in years. When she completed the Impact of Weight Worksheet, Karen realized that her weight and body image concerns have affected all aspects of her life. Karen feels ready to try a different approach. She is seeking a new family doctor whom she will feel more comfortable with so that she can get her health risks assessed. Karen also identified a number of life goals that she would like to work on, like buying new clothes that fit and beginning to date again, which would require her to become comfortable with being hugged or touched.

DO YOU HAVE AN EATING DISORDER?

People struggling with excess weight rarely think they have an eating disorder, since this is something they associate with those who are thin. However, eating disorders can affect people of any size. To determine whether you may be experiencing symptoms of an eating disorder, complete the checklist below.

Eating Disorder Behaviors Checklist

Place a check mark next to any of the following symptoms that apply to you.

- ☐ Binge eating

- ☐ Restriction of food intake or skipping meals

- ☐ Fasting (not eating for long periods)

- ☐ Behaviors to prevent weight gain after overeating (such as vomiting, using laxatives or diet pills, excessive exercise)

- ☐ Making self-worth dependent on weight and shape

- ☐ Consuming more than 25 percent of your daily calories after dinner

- ☐ Waking up from sleep to eat

If you checked off any of the symptoms above, you should see your doctor and ask to have your symptoms assessed in greater detail before you proceed further in this book. If you do have an eating disorder, you may benefit from more specialized help; weight-loss efforts may worsen an eating disorder and are not recommended. The healthy living plan discussed in this book may be helpful if you feel you have an eating disorder and would like to begin to work on recovery while you seek more specialized help. In our examples, both Karen and Jennifer show signs of an eating disorder. Karen's symptoms of regular binge eating suggest binge-eating disorder. Jennifer's eating pattern is also worrying, since she alternates between extreme calorie restriction and periods of binge eating. If this were to continue, it could develop into an eating disorder such as bulimia.

You now have a sense of the health risks associated with your current weight, and the impact your weight and body image concerns have had on your life. You are almost ready to make a change.

CHAPTER CHECKLIST

You have completed this chapter when:

○ You have calculated your BMI and WC to determine your risk of developing weight-related health problems.

○ You have seen your doctor to review and identify your weight-related health risks and complete the Medical Assessment Checklist.

○ You have set your food and activity goals for improving your health risks related to heart disease, diabetes, or cancer, if these are relevant risks for you.

○ You have calculated your realistic weight-loss goal, if any.

○ You have examined the impact that your weight has had on your life by completing the Impact of Weight Worksheet and the Worksheet Review.

○ You have completed the Eating Disorder Behaviors Checklist to determine whether you may have symptoms of an eating disorder.

What do you do next, and when?

○ Set a follow-up appointment with your doctor for six months from now to evaluate your risk factors after you have implemented your chosen weight management strategy.

○ If you checked off any of the symptoms in the Eating Disorder Behaviors Checklist, schedule an appointment with your family doctor so that you can have your symptoms assessed and determine whether you may need more specialized help.

○ After you have completed the steps above, you are ready to move on to chapter 3 and determine the best weight management approach for you.

CHAPTER 3

Making Choices: Deciding What Weight Management Approach Is Right for You

In this chapter, you will learn about various weight management options and decide on the option that best suits you.

OPTION 1: HEALTHY LIVING

The healthy living option is based on the idea that weight is strongly regulated by the body and that it's better to work *with* your own biology than against it. We know from research that people who strive to live in a healthy way and accept their "natural" weight are the most likely to be satisfied with their body, regardless of how much they weigh (Laliberte et al. 2007). Weight loss is rarely successful in the long term, so you may be better off striving for a solution that you know you can count on. Healthy living is an option for people who want to feel confident that they are living a healthy lifestyle, learn to accept themselves and be comfortable in their "natural" body, and comfortably enjoy food as part of a healthy life.

Healthy Living Option: Food

In the healthy living option, you will develop a healthy eating plan with a balanced intake of grains, fruits and vegetables, dairy, and meat or vegetarian alternatives. This plan is based on food guides accepted around the world but will be designed specifically for you. There are no "good" or "bad" foods in this plan; you will learn how to eat all foods, including "treat" foods, in a way that's healthy. Your eating will be a healthy version of what's considered "normal" in your culture and will allow you to comfortably take part in social occasions. You will also be able to have a couple of special-occasion meals each week that include rich or plentiful food.

Healthy Living Option: Activity

In the healthy living option, you will regularly include physical activity in your life. This may be structured, planned exercise that you set time aside for on a regular basis, or it may be activity that you gradually build into your life. You will choose one or more activities that are consistent with your current interests and priorities.

Putting the Healthy Living Option into Practice

How will you change your old patterns to new ones? Changing your lifestyle will take time. We will offer you numerous suggestions, based on our experience working with people making these changes to their lifestyles. But, most important, we are going to help you figure out what is getting in your way. Each bump in the road will be an opportunity to understand what went wrong and to put a solution in place so that eventually you will follow your plan with ease.

Healthy Living Option: Body Image

The first step toward feeling good about your body is to feel confident that you are living a healthy lifestyle, as we just discussed. The next step is to directly target the thoughts and behaviors that fuel body dissatisfaction. In the chapters on body image, you will learn strategies that help people feel more satisfied with their bodies.

Who Is Suited to the Healthy Living Option?

The healthy living option is recommended for people who fall within the "healthy" or "overweight" BMI range and who don't currently have any pressing weight-related medical concerns. If this describes you and your main reason for wanting to lose weight is that you are unhappy with your appearance, then this option might be for you. This is also the option we would recommend for anyone who is struggling with binge eating. Learning to eat in a regular, healthy way will prevent further weight gain. Feeling in control of your eating and regularly meeting your body's needs will also go a long way toward improving your emotional well-being. Even if you ultimately consider one of the other weight loss options, starting from a base of regular, healthy eating is more likely to make you successful.

The healthy living option may also be recommended if you have tried such options as surgery or medication but have nonetheless regained your weight, especially if you have had difficulty with binge eating or losing control of your eating.

Is the Healthy Living Option a Possibility for You?

STEP 1: Do any of the following statements apply to you? Check all that apply.

☐ I am sick of yo-yo dieting.

☐ I want to be able to enjoy my food but also live a more healthy life.

☐ I want to be able to eat all foods in a healthy way.

☐ I am willing to increase my activity level as part of my daily life.

☐ I am willing to see where my "natural" weight will be.

☐ I am open to working on my body dissatisfaction and learning to be more comfortable with my size.

☐ My BMI is less than 30, or if it is above 30, I have no medical problems.

☐ I do not have any pressing medical concerns related to my weight.

☐ I have problems with binge eating.

☐ I have tried surgery or medication to control my weight but have regained any weight that I lost.

☐ I want to prepare for weight-loss surgery.

STEP 2: Consider the healthy living option.

- Normalized eating
  - regular meals and snacks
  - variety of foods
- Gradual addition of physical activity

PROS

- This is not a restrictive diet. You can eat moderately from a wide variety of foods.
- The plan is based on recommendations for good health.
- You can trust your weight to be stable rather than undergoing the ups and downs of a life of dieting.
- Working on body image can address body dissatisfaction in a more lasting way than weight loss can.

CONS

- Although eating is flexible, this option still requires planning and structure for your meals.
- This is a harder option to accept if you have had your heart set on weight loss.

OPTION 2: WEIGHT LOSS THROUGH LIFESTYLE CHANGES

The option of weight loss through lifestyle changes is based on the idea that modest weight loss can lead to significant health and body image improvements. Just 5 to 15 percent of your body weight is a realistic amount to aim for. It's also important to be realistic about what is required to lose weight and maintain that weight loss. Gradual weight loss is the safest and most long-lasting approach. This is a permanent lifestyle change, not a quick fix. It's similar to the healthy living option reviewed previously, but more intensive; food intake is more restricted, the exercise is more intense, and weight monitoring is done on a daily or weekly basis. This approach can also include body image work, which research suggests may help to maintain weight loss, and the use of medication (see option 3).

Weight Loss Through Lifestyle Changes: Food

In this approach, you will follow what's called a "balanced deficit plan." We will calculate the calories you need in order to maintain your current weight, and we will reduce that amount by five hundred calories per day. You will develop a balanced and low-fat meal plan based on this target. We encourage you to make high-fiber grain choices, as this will help to keep you satisfied for longer. We discourage you from drinking alcoholic beverages, partly because of the calories in these drinks and partly because they may make you more likely to overeat. You won't need special foods on this plan, although you may find it easier to stick to your plan if you don't allow yourself too many options.

Weight Loss Through Lifestyle Changes: Activity

With this approach, you will *eventually* be doing one hour of vigorous activity per day, six days per week. This amount of activity is based on what we know about the activity levels of successful weight losers—the majority of whom choose to walk daily, most walking for about one hour. The activity you choose should be based on both what's physically comfortable for you and what you can see yourself sustaining in the long run. Finding a partner to join you in your activity will likely help with motivation, and having goals to work toward (like participating in a yearly walk for charity) can enhance your sense of accomplishment.

Putting the Weight Loss Through Lifestyle Changes Option into Practice

How will you change your old patterns and adopt new ones? As is the case with the healthy living option, you will start by planning and then move toward your planned lifestyle. We will provide you with general guidelines that have been shown to help people to successfully follow a weight loss meal plan. We will also help you to identify the specific "bumps in the road" that put you at risk for falling off your plan. We will suggest strategies for managing risky situations, emotions that trigger overeating, and interactions that may upset you. We suggest that you find a support network for individuals trying to lose weight, and someone (a friend, family member, or therapist) you can check in with on a weekly basis to review difficulties that come up and listen to your plans for solving these problems.

Weight Loss Through Lifestyle Changes: Body Image

You may be planning to lose weight in order to feel better about your body. It likely *will* make you feel better, even the modest weight loss that we are recommending. However, people who rely on weight loss to feel better about their body are very vulnerable to feeling dissatisfied if they regain even a small amount of weight. Even if weight loss does improve your body satisfaction, you will likely still experience some dissatisfaction. We therefore recommend that you also plan to complete the body image section of this workbook.

Who Is Suited to the Weight Loss Through Lifestyle Changes Option?

This option is recommended if you are overweight or obese. It is not recommended if you are in the "healthy" weight range. If your BMI is greater than 40, or if you are experiencing weight-related health problems, you may want to talk with your physician about more intensive weight-loss options (such as medication and surgery; see option 3). The weight loss through lifestyle changes option is also recommended if you know that you are organized and disciplined, and believe that you can follow a plan consistently. It is not recommended if you have a tendency to become overly restrictive in your eating or if you tend to overdo your physical activity. In addition, this option is not recommended as the only strategy for managing body image concerns. If the way you feel about your body is what bothers you most, then we recommend that you use the body image section (see chapters 10 and 11) as your main strategy.

Is the Weight Loss Through Lifestyle Changes Option a Possibility for You?

STEP 1: Do any of the following statements apply to you? Check all that apply.

☐ I would like to lose weight so that I am healthier.

☐ I am ready to make permanent changes to my lifestyle.

☐ I am prepared to do the work needed to maintain these changes.

☐ I am open to planning and following a meal plan.

☐ I am willing to build exercise into my life on a regular basis.

☐ My BMI is greater than 25.

☐ I do not have eating disorder symptoms (problems with binge eating, restricting, and so on).

☐ I am considering taking weight loss medication.

STEP 2: Consider the Weight Loss Through Lifestyle Changes Option

■ Gradual long-term sustainable changes to your eating plan

■ Addition of regular physical activity

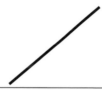

PROS

■ The food plan you develop is one you can follow over your lifetime. It allows you to develop new habits.

■ You may benefit from having scheduled and limited choices, which can prevent you from overeating.

■ Physical activity as part of your daily life can not only help you manage your weight but also boost your mood and energy levels.

CONS

■ You will need to plan for social events to make sure you can stick with your plan. Relaxed overeating will keep you from losing or maintaining your weight loss.

■ Weight loss occurs more slowly than in more extreme or restrictive diets; you need to take a long-term perspective and evaluate changes over months, not weeks. But remember, this is meant to last a lifetime!

■ Structured eating can feel restrictive and frustrating at times.

OPTION 3: WEIGHT LOSS SUPPORTED BY MEDICATION

The option of adding medication to a weight-loss effort is based on the understanding that weight is biologically regulated, and to successfully maintain weight loss, some people need a biologically based intervention. With this option, you follow the weight-loss plan to limit your eating, and you are also encouraged to be physically active. The research clearly shows that, without these lifestyle changes, medication is not successful. Because medications can sometimes have side effects (described later), we would recommend that you try them only after trying to lose weight through lifestyle changes. However, medication will make it easier to maintain the more restricted eating necessary for weight loss.

Obesity is best understood as a chronic illness, like diabetes or high blood pressure, which may require medication. For example, if a person with high blood pressure stops taking her medication, her blood pressure can be expected to go back up to unhealthy levels. Similarly, weight-loss medications may help you lose weight and maintain that lower weight, but if the medications are discontinued, you will regain the weight you have lost. Note that we don't yet have the research to understand how these medications work over the long term. It's possible, therefore, that at some point you may need to make changes to your medication regimen or stop taking the medication altogether.

Medication Option: Food

It would be nice if you could take a medication and continue to eat as decadently as you like. Unfortunately, medications don't work this way. To successfully lose weight and maintain that weight loss, you need to make the same changes to your lifestyle that you would if you were trying to lose weight without medication. The difference is that medication will make it easier for you to adhere to your eating plan, or it will make weight loss easier. With medications that reduce appetite (such as Meridia), we would recommend that you follow the weight loss through lifestyle food plan (option 2). With medications that prevent absorption of certain nutrients (such as Xenical), we recommend that you follow the healthy living plan (option 1).

Medication Option: Activity

While taking medication, you need to be physically active in order to achieve and maintain weight loss. You can follow the healthy living activity plan, which allows you to set time aside for activity, or build it into your daily lifestyle.

Putting the Medication Option into Practice

This option requires that you work closely with your physician. If your doctor feels that you are a candidate for medication, and she prescribes medication for you, you will need to be monitored for side effects. See the following table for a brief description of the medications and possible side effects.

Drug	Trade Name	How It Works	Common Side Effects
Orlistat*	Xenical	Reduces fat absorption in the intestines	Abdominal bloating, pain and cramping, fecal incontinence
Alli	Xenical (reduced strength)	Reduces fat absorption in the intestines	Same as above
Sibutramine*	Meridia	Suppresses appetite	Dry mouth, constipation, dizziness
Diethylpropion	Tenuate	Suppresses appetite	Chest pain, heart palpitations
Phentermine	Adipex Inonamine SR	Suppresses appetite	Anxiety, headache, dizziness, dry mouth

*Also approved in Canada

Because this option requires that you make changes to your lifestyle, you will benefit from also reading the sections in this book that are intended to help you put the changes into practice and overcome obstacles that get in the way of change.

Medication Option: Body Image

Medications are not recommended in order to improve body image alone. They are only recommended in order to address health concerns related to excess weight. Nonetheless, as is the case with the weight loss through lifestyle changes approach (option 2), you can expect that weight loss will contribute to better body image. One of the advantages of taking medication is that you can be more certain of maintaining your weight loss. However, you are still looking at a weight loss of only 5 to 15 percent of your body weight. Although this amount of weight loss is associated with significant improvements in body image, you will likely still have some areas of dissatisfaction. We recommend that you work through the body image chapters in this book in order to manage your dissatisfaction.

Who Is Suited to the Medication Option?

This option is recommended for you if your weight falls in the obese range or if you are experiencing health concerns related to being overweight. Improving your health or reducing the risk of disease should be the primary goals for treatment. Your doctor will have to agree that medications would be helpful in this regard. This option is not recommended for people who are slightly overweight. It is also not recommended for the purpose of improving body image. Depending upon your particular medical profile, your physician may decide that you cannot safely take certain medications. You must also be monitored after you start taking medication to be sure there are no troubling side effects.

Is the Medication Option a Possibility for You?

STEP 1: Do any of the following statements apply to you? Check all that apply.

☐ My BMI is greater than 40.

☐ My BMI is over 30 and I have health risk factors because of my weight.

☐ My waist circumference is greater than 88 cm. or 35 in. (female).

☐ My waist circumference is greater than 102 cm. or 40 in. (male).

☐ I am not solely interested in improving my body image.

☐ I would like help with following a weight loss through lifestyle changes plan.

STEP 2: Consider the Medication Option.

■ Medication is added to support efforts at weight loss through lifestyle changes.

PROS

■ The use of medication to help control weight can make weight loss and the maintenance of weight loss easier.

■ The changes in diet required while taking medication can help you develop healthy eating habits.

■ The medication can help you get your weight down to a level at which physical activity becomes more reasonable.

CONS

■ Not all medications are safe for everyone. Check with your doctor.

■ Medications can have side effects. You will have to evaluate your own reaction to the medication you try.

■ Not everyone feels comfortable with the idea of taking a medication over the long term.

■ This approach still requires that you make changes to your eating habits and activity levels in order to maximize success.

OPTION 4: WEIGHT LOSS (BARIATRIC) SURGERY

Weight loss (bariatric) surgery is reserved for people who are either severely overweight (with a BMI over 40), or who have a BMI over 35 and have weight-related health problems. Bariatric surgery involves the modification of your digestive system to limit the amount of food you can consume, limit the absorption of nutrients through your intestine, or both. The two most common bariatric surgery procedures are gastric bypass and adjustable gastric banding. Gastric bypass surgery reduces the size of your stomach to that of a small pouch connected directly to the small intestine so that food "bypasses" a large portion of the stomach and part of your small intestine. In adjustable gastric banding, small incisions or holes are made laproscopically and an adjustable gastric band is placed around an area of your stomach to limit the size of the stomach and control the amount of food that enters your intestine. The size of the food passage can be increased or decreased by adjusting the tightness of the band.

Bariatric surgery is a treatment specifically meant to reduce the health risks and problems associated with obesity. The option of surgery is based on the understanding that weight is biologically regulated, and that when significant weight loss is required for medical reasons, it is not likely to be maintained through lifestyle changes alone. It's also based on the understanding of obesity as a chronic illness that requires, in some circumstances, more invasive treatment. Weight-loss surgery is only recommended when other weight loss options have failed. There are risks associated with surgery, so we strongly recommend that you choose a facility staffed by people with many years of experience with bariatric surgery. We also recommend that you arrange for medical (and ideally, nutritional) follow-up after your surgery, particularly if you live far away from the surgery facility. Medical monitoring will be necessary throughout the remainder of your life.

Surgery Option: Food

As is the case with the medication option previously described, weight loss through surgery does not occur by magic. The purpose of surgery is to change the mechanics of your digestive system so that you are forced to eat very small amounts of food. As a result, even a small amount of food should leave you feeling very full.

Your eating plan after weight-loss surgery will consist primarily of low-fat proteins (lean meats such as chicken, turkey, and fish), fruits, and vegetables. But *how* you eat will change just as much as *what* you eat. Meal portions must be small, you must eat slowly, and food must be chewed thoroughly. If you eat too much, eat too fast, or don't completely chew your food, you may experience nausea or vomiting. You will have to avoid drinking liquids with meals, or just before or after meals, since liquids could force food through your stomach pouch too quickly. This may cause you to become hungry during the day or may cause you to feel ill and have diarrhea. You will need to schedule three regular mealtimes per day, and eat only at those scheduled mealtimes. You should not skip meals, nor should you snack between meals. When you feel full, you will have to stop eating. Overeating can not only cause nausea and vomiting but can also stretch out your stomach pouch. When you first start on your solid diet, you may only be able to eat four to six bites of food before you feel full. With time, you may be able to eat a half cup to one cup of food; eventually you will be able to consume an amount of food that's typical for successful long-term weight losers (about thirteen hundred calories per day). Because of the changes to your eating habits that occur with different types of surgery, you may need to take nutritional supplements. Check with a dietitian or your follow-up care provider.

Surgery Option: Activity

As is the case with all the weight-loss options, physical activity is recommended as a part of your long-term plan. As with any surgery, you will need your physician's permission to start physical activity; once you have the green light, you will be encouraged to follow a plan similar to that for the healthy living option discussed previously.

Putting the Surgery Option into Practice

With this option, you will work closely with your physician to decide whether surgery is appropriate for you. You will also need to be monitored by a physician following surgery to ensure that you are recovering and adjusting properly. Ideally, you will participate in a comprehensive program staffed by a variety of health care professionals, including a dietitian from whom you can get nutritional advice. Prior to surgery, try the healthy living option (option 1) so that you develop regular, scheduled eating habits. Starting the restrictive and structured eating patterns required after surgery is much more overwhelming if your eating has been very chaotic prior to the surgery. We would therefore recommend that you read the chapters devoted to helping you adopt more normalized eating habits and moderate physical activity. We also recommend that you work through the chapters on body image. As discussed below, surgery results in a tremendous amount of weight loss, which has a significant impact on body image. However, weight regain is common after the second or third year, and there may still be issues of body dissatisfaction, despite weight loss.

Surgery Option: Body Image

Bariatric surgery results in at least a 50 percent loss of excess body weight when a patient is compliant with the protocol and receives multidisciplinary care. This type of dramatic change in appearance will almost certainly have a positive impact on your body image (van Hout et al. 2008). Often the massive weight loss is accompanied by other problems, however, the most dramatic of which, for some people, is an excessive amount of loose skin. This problem can be so bothersome for people that they require cosmetic body-contouring surgery. It would be important for you to fully discuss these issues with your physician, and perhaps with a support group made up of people who have had weight-loss surgery, before choosing to undergo this procedure (Sarwer et al. 2008). Because body image concerns can emerge after surgery despite the positive impact of weight loss, we recommend that you work through the body image chapters as you go through this process.

Who Is Suited to the Weight-Loss Surgery Option?

Weight-loss surgery is the most extreme of the interventions we list here. It's also the treatment that provides the most dramatic results, with significant improvement to weight-related health concerns and body image. This treatment is not for everyone, however, and it's important that you have a thorough physical and psychological assessment prior to having this procedure. Weight-loss surgery may not be an effective or safe option for those with too low BMI (less than 32), heart attack or stroke within the previous six months, and less than 5 years after treatment for certain cancers (Yermilov, McGory, Shekelle, Ko, and Maggard 2009). In addition, surgery is not appropriate for individuals with severe untreated mental illness, active suicidal thoughts, current bulimia or active purging, and current substance abuse (Fabricatore et al. 2006). Other weight management strategies should be pursued while these issues are properly addressed.

Weight-loss surgery has been found to be successful even for people with problems with binge eating. However, in these cases, adjustable gastric banding is not recommended, because long-term studies show that people who have struggled with binge eating tend to develop another type of eating disorder after surgery, in which they deliberately eat to the point of throwing up. Even though the amount of food eaten is actually quite small, the loss of control is associated with significant weight regain (for review see Mitchell et al. 2006). Our experience has been that people who binge-eat do particularly well with bypass surgery if they first work to stabilize their food intake and overcome their binge eating.

Is the Weight-Loss Surgery Option a Possibility for You?

STEP 1: Do any of the following statements apply to you? Check all that apply.

☐ My BMI is greater than 40.

☐ My BMI is over 35 and I have health complications because of my weight.

☐ I have tried other weight-loss approaches without success.

☐ I have discussed medication with my physician.

☐ I believe the risks of surgery are worth taking to overcome the risks of my weight.

☐ I understand that I will need to be medically supported and monitored after my surgery.

☐ I do not have problems with substance abuse.

☐ I do not have problems with binge eating.

☐ I am not solely interested in improving my body image.

STEP 2: Consider the Weight-Loss Surgery Option.

■ Your digestive system is surgically altered so that you are forced to eat very small amounts of food.

PROS

■ This option can result in rapid, large amounts of weight loss.

■ It supports any changes you make to your eating by controlling your appetite.

■ It can help you reach a weight where you can become physically active more easily.

CONS

■ There are risks associated with surgery.

■ You will need to make drastic changes to what foods and how much you eat.

■ You will require lifelong medical monitoring.

■ Finding the medical, nutritional, and emotional support you will need may be difficult for those who live in certain geographic areas.

Choosing Your Weight Management Approach

After reading through the decision trees and considering the pros and cons for each weight-loss option, do you know which weight management option you will choose? If so, write it below:

_____

_____

If you are considering the medication or surgery options, you will need to consult with your doctor before you proceed. However, you can still get started with either the healthy living or the weight loss through lifestyle changes options, because they will help you prepare in the meantime. If you have an eating disorder, then the weight-loss options are *not* recommended and could lead to worsening of your symptoms; see your family doctor to assess your need for more specialized help, and consider trying the healthy living option.

Jim liked the description of the healthy living option, but he didn't feel that he had the choice of "accepting" his weight. He was experiencing significant weight-related health problems and his physician recommended weight loss. He wasn't sure that medication was the best option, because he might not lose enough weight to help with his mobility problems. He was seriously considering the bariatric surgery option, specifically adjustable gastric banding. In the meantime, he thought he would try the balanced deficit weight loss plan to improve his eating before surgery.

Karen also felt that she really didn't have the option of accepting her weight. Like Jim, she had health concerns related to her weight and she was very unhappy with her appearance. She wanted to lose weight, but her bingeing was out of control. She knew that if she didn't control her binge eating, her weight would just keep climbing. She decided that this would be her priority for now. She would try the healthy living approach, since this was recommended for stopping binge eating. When her binge eating was under control, she would consider other options.

The healthy living option also appealed to Janice, as she was already trying to make healthy choices when she was at home. However, with her weight falling just in the obese range, she was still interested in the weight-loss option. She wasn't sure that she wanted to add medication into the picture until she had tried making lifestyle changes on her own. Janice typically succeeded when she put her mind to something, so she felt that she could manage a moderate weight loss approach. Her father's heart attack had frightened her, and she had already decided that she needed to become more active. Janice had the financial means to join a fitness club and knew that she could stay in hotels with fitness facilities when she traveled for work. She wanted to try the weight loss through lifestyle changes option.

Carlos thought the healthy living option sounded great. He really couldn't imagine living a restrictive lifestyle—he liked socializing and eating too much. But he was prepared to try to make sensible changes to his eating during the week. Also, he quite liked the idea of becoming more active again. He planned to talk with his doctor to see whether she would recommend weight loss medications in addition to the medications he had been prescribed for his cholesterol and blood pressure.

Jennifer realized that the healthy living option was really the only one recommended for her. She was having some difficulty giving up on her dreams of weight loss, but she found that the notion that her body regulated her weight made perfect sense. She could see that the only way she could maintain a lower weight was by starving, even though other people of her height seemed to maintain this lower weight without difficulty. The idea that she just had different genetics made sense to her, especially as her sister also seemed to have the same body type. Jennifer's weight loss never seemed to last, and she was miserable with her body when she regained her weight. Maybe working toward a healthy lifestyle and better body image was worth a shot.

What if I Don't Feel Ready to Commit to an Approach?

At this point, you may feel ready to dive right in and get started. Or, you may be unsure and not quite ready to commit. It's completely normal to feel hesitant about making changes in your life. After all, you may have had many experiences where you tried to make changes and didn't experience any benefits. It wouldn't be surprising if you had feelings of helplessness, hopelessness, or skepticism about another attempt at change. In the next chapter, we will guide you through some exercises that will help you to explore any ambivalence you may have about embarking on a new weight management approach. This process will help you to feel more ready to commit to the strategy that best suits you.

CHAPTER CHECKLIST

You have successfully completed this chapter when:

O   You have worked through the decision tree for each approach to determine which approaches would be options for you.

O   You have considered the pros and cons of each of the approaches and identified the weight management option that's the best fit for you.

What do you do next and when?

O   If you have decided on a medication or surgery option, sct up an appointment with your family doctor to find out more information and discuss the suitability of the approach for you from a medical perspective.

O   After you have completed the steps above, you are ready to move on to chapter 4 and begin preparing for your change journey.

Making Preparations: Getting Ready for Your Change Journey

You have identified a weight-management approach that suits you. But are you *really* ready to make the necessary changes to your lifestyle? This chapter will help enhance your motivation and ensure that you mobilize your support systems in order to maximize your success on this journey.

INCREASING YOUR READINESS TO MAKE CHANGES

According to the transtheoretical model of change (Prochaska, Norcross, and DiClemente 1994), people move toward making changes to their behavior by going through a series of stages of readiness:

1. **Precontemplation** ("I don't think I have a problem and I don't need to change.")

2. **Contemplation** ("I realize I have a problem and I am thinking about making changes, but I haven't completely decided.")

3. **Preparation** ("I intend to do something about my problem and I am just getting ready.")

4. **Action** ("I am ready and have even started to make changes in my life.")

5. **Maintenance** ("I want to continue the changes that I have made so that they are long lasting.")

Because you are reading this book, we can guess that you are at least in the contemplation stage of readiness. You would like to make some changes in your life related to your eating and activity patterns, but you may or may not feel entirely ready to do so. If you are in the preparation stage, you are planning to make changes and you probably hope that this book will guide you along. If you are in the action phase, you are ready to jump right in and may have already started to make changes. It's important to examine readiness for change, because it has been found to predict positive outcomes in treatment programs (DiClemente and Velasquez 2002). Our goal is to help you move you into the action stage using strategies designed to enhance motivation (Miller and Rollnick 2002).

How Ready Are You to Make a Change?

Using the scale below, rate how ready you feel to start on your change journey using the weight-management strategy you selected in chapter 3.

0% --100%

Not at All   Extremely
Ready   Ready

I am _____% ready.

If your rating is 80 percent or above, you are in action mode and are well motivated to get started. If your rating is between 60 and 80 percent, then you have a bit of work to do before you start. If your rating is less than 60 percent, then you need to figure out what factors are keeping that rating from being higher. Regardless of your actual readiness rating, the exercises in this chapter will help you to boost your motivation and reduce your ambivalence about making changes to your eating, activity, and lifestyle. You can start by answering the questions below to understand your readiness rating:

1. What factors or concerns keep this percentage from being higher? Also, consider practical factors that might make it difficult for you to make changes at this time (such as work-related stress, school schedule, and so on).

    _____

    _____

2. What factors keep this percentage from being lower? What hopes and expectations are pushing you forward? What are your reasons to change?

    _____

    _____

3. Do you have specific concerns about trying the weight management strategy that best suits you?

_____

_____

4. What have you learned from prior change attempts? What worked or didn't work?

_____

_____

Janice rated her readiness to try the weight loss through lifestyle changes option at 65 percent. She didn't rate it higher because she's not sure she will be able to make the changes needed when she's traveling. When she stays in hotels, she rewards herself by eating decadently, and going to the hotel gym after a long day at conferences seems difficult. However, Janice is really concerned about her health, especially her heart, and she feels she owes it to her kids to try making changes.

Janice's main concern is how she will find the time in her busy travel schedule to plan physical activity and incorporate healthy meals.

Shifting the Balance of Change

Before completing the exercise above, you may have already been aware of the reasons to implement a weight management approach and make changes in your life. You may have been less aware of your reasons for *not* changing. It's these hidden reasons, the costs of change, that often keep you from moving ahead with your goals. If you understand your obstacles, you can address them so that they are less likely to block your path. To have a clear understanding of your reasons for and against change, complete the Cost-Benefit Analysis Worksheet, which follows. To help you see how to do this, we have provided Janice's worksheet as an example.

Janice's Cost-Benefit Analysis Worksheet

Reflect on the costs and benefits associated with making a change or keeping things the same. *Consider both the short-term and long-term impact on your life.* Write the costs and benefits in the corresponding boxes below. Beside each one, rate how important you think that cost or benefit is, from 0 (not at all) to 100 (extremely).

MOVING FORWARD WITH CHANGE AND IMPLEMENTING A WEIGHT-MANAGEMENT APPROACH

SHORT-TERM COSTS

- *It won't be fun to cut back my eating. 80*
- *It will be hard to find time to exercise when I don't feel like it. 60*
- *I am worried I will get depressed if I can't enjoy my food when I am away from my family. 90*
- *It will interfere with my social life, because I won't be able to enjoy dinner parties in the same way. 70*

SHORT-TERM BENEFITS

- *I will feel like I am getting healthier. 90*
- *I will feel more in control of my life. 80*
- *Exercise may help me relieve stress and sleep better. 50*
- *I can feel closer to my husband if we do this together. 60*
- *I might meet people and have fun if I join a fitness club. 40*
- *I will feel better about my body. 80*

LONG-TERM COSTS

- *I might fail in this approach and then feel bad about myself. 90*
- *I will lose the freedom of not having to think about food or exercise. 90*

LONG-TERM BENEFITS

- *My physical health will improve. 100*
- *I will lower my risk of heart disease. 100*
- *I will be around longer to enjoy life and be there for my kids. 100*
- *I will enjoy my life more if I am feeling healthier and strong. 80*
- *I will feel more satisfied with my appearance. 80*
- *It will help me to make myself a priority in my life. 70*

STAYING WHERE YOU ARE AND NOT MAKING ANY CHANGES

SHORT-TERM COSTS

- I won't feel good about myself if I am not trying to become healthier. 70
- My physical health is at risk with my current lifestyle. 80
- I am unhappy with my appearance. 60

SHORT-TERM BENEFITS

- It is easier. 90
- I can eat what I want. 90
- I can reward myself with food. 80
- I can socialize around food events with freedom. 70
- I don't have to find energy to exercise. 60
- I won't have to find time in my schedule for planning. 70

LONG-TERM COSTS

- I am compromising my physical health. 80
- I am at risk of heart disease. 90
- I may not live as long and be there for my kids. 100
- I will feel like I didn't give myself the effort that I deserve. 60
- I will continue to feel dissatisfied with my body. 60
- I will have less energy. 50

LONG-TERM BENEFITS

- I won't have to think about my eating or how much I exercise. 80
- I can just live my life as I have always done. 70
- I won't set myself up for failure. You can't fail if you don't try. 60

Cost-Benefit Analysis Worksheet

Reflect on the costs and benefits associated with making a change or staying the same. *Consider both the short-term and long-term impact on your life.* Write the costs and benefits in the corresponding boxes below. Beside each one, rate how important you think that cost or benefit is, from 0 (not at all) to 100 (extremely).

MOVING FORWARD WITH CHANGE AND IMPLEMENTING A WEIGHT-MANAGEMENT APPROACH

SHORT-TERM COSTS	**SHORT-TERM BENEFITS**

LONG-TERM COSTS	**LONG-TERM BENEFITS**

STAYING WHERE YOU ARE AND NOT MAKING ANY CHANGES

SHORT-TERM COSTS	SHORT-TERM BENEFITS

LONG-TERM COSTS	LONG-TERM BENEFITS

Learning from the Costs and Benefits

Now that you have thought through the costs and benefits of changing your lifestyle, let's reflect on what you have discovered:

1. When you consider the costs and benefits of *changing,* do you notice that one list is longer than the other? Are there specific costs or benefits that you rated as particularly important to you? If so, what are they? Which list seems more compelling?

   _____

   _____

2. When you examine the costs of making a change, do you see ways you can overcome these drawbacks? Resolve each cost below if you can. Ask your partner or a friend for ideas of ways to deal with the costs.

   _____

   _____

   _____

3. When you consider the costs and benefits of *staying the same,* do you notice that one list is longer than the other? Are there specific costs or benefits that you rated as particularly important to you? If so, what are they? On the balance, which list seems more compelling?

   _____

   _____

   _____

4. When you examine the benefits of staying the same, can you see ways that you might find these same benefits through different methods? For example, if a benefit of staying the same is that you have a way of coping with your emotions, could you set a goal to find other ways of coping with emotions?

   _____

   _____

   _____

We hope that exploring the costs and benefits of moving forward with change and with staying the same has given you some clarity about whether you are ready to commit to change. Before you make your decision, we also want to look at your thoughts and beliefs, both about your capacity to make changes and the faith you have in the plan you are considering.

Is Your Head in the Right Place?

The weight management approaches that we are advocating are not diets or temporary lifestyle changes; rather, they are permanent lifestyle changes that you will implement as a new way of life. This is your opportunity to shed the old habits and embark on a new you! Even as you are reading this, you are probably thinking negative and skeptical thoughts ("Yeah, right. Like this is going to work. I have been through this so many times before."). These thoughts are common, but if you don't address them, they can get in the way of your success. So let's pull out those thoughts and put them right on the table.

STEP 1

Make a list of your negative thoughts about starting a weight management approach in the left column of the following box. The thoughts might be about the approach itself, or about your capacity to carry out the approach.

STEP 2

For each negative thought, come up with a response that counters that point and write it in the right column. Imagine that you are a lawyer trying to provide evidence from the other side. What would you say? Or, consider what a friend would say if you told him your negative thought. In the following table, we have filled in a few examples.

Negative Thoughts	Countering Thought
"Yeah, right. Like this is going to work."	"Well, I won't know unless I try. What do I have to lose? It's not like I am happy right now, anyway."
"I have been through this so many times before."	"This is a different approach. It's not another diet. It's about making permanent changes that I can sustain. These plans seem more realistic."
"I won't be able to cope if I can't use my eating to make me feel better."	"I will learn new ways of coping and managing my emotions. It just may take more time."

Now that we have explored any ambivalence you may have about embarking on a new weight management approach, it's time to rerate your readiness to change.

Using the scale below, rate how ready you feel to start on your change journey.

0% --100%

Not at All   Extremely
Ready   Ready

I am _____% ready.

We hope these exercises have helped you to realistically evaluate whether this is the right time to start making a significant lifestyle change. If your rating has moved close to 80 percent or above, you are ready to move into the action stage. If your readiness rating continues to be 60 percent or lower, then we hope that you have uncovered some of the reasons for your reluctance to change in this chapter. You may need to address some of the practical and emotional obstacles before you begin making changes. It's better to choose the right time to begin change rather than start down this path when you are unlikely to be successful.

When you are ready to begin, we recommend that you make a commitment for at least six months. This time frame gives you the opportunity to give it a try and see the effects on your weight, health risks, and well-being.

In the space below, write in the approach that you will follow:

I commit to following the _____ approach for six months.

Are Your Support Systems Ready?

As you have learned, successfully managing your weight will require a permanent change in your lifestyle, regardless of the approach you choose. As is the case with most big projects, your chances of success are much better when you have a good support system.

Janice is planning to hire a personal trainer to help motivate her to exercise, as well as teach her an exercise routine that she can use at home and when she travels for work. Janice's husband has agreed to be her exercise partner so that they can support each other and work out together. Janice has also found a great online support group, so she has access to friends who can help her when she travels.

MEDICAL AND PROFESSIONAL SUPPORT

Your doctor is an essential part of your weight management support system. In particular, your doctor is responsible for assessing and helping you manage the health risks associated with being overweight or obese. You doctor will also monitor the impact of your lifestyle changes on your risk factors over time. Regularly checking in with a health care professional—particularly one who can offer you advice when you face difficulties—has also been shown to help people stay on track once they have made changes to their eating and activity (Perri et al. 1984). The weight management approaches described in this book have been specifically chosen because they are unlikely to result in medical complications. If you choose weight-loss medication or surgery, however, close monitoring of your health by your physician is essential. Before you begin your weight management plan, meet with your doctor to describe your plans and seek her input.

Now, describe your professional supports below:

My Medical and Professional Supports (for example, family doctor, dietitian, therapist, personal trainer):

_____

YOUR SOCIAL CONTEXT

Social support has been shown to be important in the process of achieving and maintaining changes in health behavior. Health professionals, family members, friends, work colleagues, church communities, and social organizations may all be part of your natural support network and can play a role in helping with your weight management. However, just as your support network can help you to achieve your goals, their lack of support can be a significant barrier to your success. Before you embark on your weight management plan, talk with family, friends, and coworkers and elicit their support. Finding new sources of support, such as weight-loss groups or online chat forums, may also be helpful if you feel you need more support than is available to you in your social network (Helgeson and Gottlieb 2000).

Identify your personal and organization supports below:

My Personal Supports (for example, close friends, family members, work colleagues)

_____

My Organization Supports (for example, online support group, weight-loss support group, health club, exercise club)

_____

Tips for Family Members and Friends

Below is a list of tips that may be useful to share with those supporting you as you implement changes for managing your weight.

- Help your loved one eat healthier: provide healthier food choices at home or work, offer social activities that don't always include eating out, and help try to establish routine eating habits.

- Acknowledge that making lifestyle changes is a challenge. Help remind your loved one that the changes are for a lifetime, and be patient with him.

- Get involved: it's often easier to overcome obstacles with a partner. When possible, join a gym together or make the same changes yourself.

- Don't become a food cop! What you see as support, your loved one may see as harassment.

- Don't make it difficult for your loved one to follow her plan. For example, if you want to snack on foods that your loved one has had problems eating in a controlled way, ask how you can do this without creating more difficulties.

- Don't feel threatened when your loved one is successful. A physical change doesn't change who your loved one is, or how important you are to your loved one.

- Don't emphasize failure. It's not uncommon to "fall off the wagon" and have a setback. This does not mean all is lost. Remember, "I told you so" is not helpful or appreciated!

CHAPTER CHECKLIST

You have successfully completed this chapter when:

O You have examined the factors that have influenced your "readiness to change" rating.

O You have worked through the Cost-Benefit Analysis Worksheet and reflected on how these factors influence your readiness to change.

O You have examined and challenged the negative thoughts that stand in your way.

O You have made a commitment to follow the weight management approach that's the best fit for you for the next six months. Or, you have decided to focus on overcoming the obstacles to change before making a commitment to change.

O You have identified your support systems.

What do you do next, and when?

O If you have not yet done so, engage your medical support systems by making an appointment with your family doctor and discussing your plan.

O Mobilize your social supports. Discuss what you are doing and how your friends and relatives can help you.

O After you have completed the steps above, you are ready to move on to chapter 5 and develop your personalized eating plan.

Changing Your Lifestyle: Designing Your Eating Plan

It's time to get to work. In this chapter, we will work out the details of your weight management approach and, in particular, what you will eat. The plan will be tailored for you based on the weight management approach you have selected. It is very important to note that if you have *already* undergone weight-loss surgery, this chapter does not apply to you. You should follow the meal plan prescribed to you by your doctor. If you find it helpful, you can monitor your progress in following your prescribed plan by using the tracking sheet at the end of the chapter and then move directly to chapter 6.

BEGINNING WITH THE BASICS

Regardless of your past experiences with managing your weight, it would not be surprising if you felt uncertain about what you should eat. The explosion of nutritional advice and diet plans in the last few decades would leave most people uncertain about the "right way" to eat or to manage their weight. The good news is that you don't need to be a nutritional expert to make good choices. Instead, you need to remember what you likely learned about eating as a child: eat balanced meals, eat at regular intervals, and enjoy treats occasionally. It's not complicated; it's a lot like the way you might feed a ten-year-old who came to visit for the day. We are going to help you tailor a plan just for you, but this plan will be built around the basics you already know.

Your Plan: Calculating Your Energy Needs

Intuitively, we all know that some people need to eat more than others. Men need to eat more than women. Young people need to eat more than older people. Tall people need to eat more than short people. Active people need to eat more than inactive people. We need to take these factors into account to figure out what your energy needs are and to plan how much you will need to eat in a day. Your energy needs determine the amount by which you will need to reduce your food intake to lose weight safely and maintain long-term weight loss.

To calculate your energy needs, we will use a well-established formula used by dietitians (Harris and Benedict 1918). We will show you Carlos's calculations as an example, and then we will show you his and Janice's eating plans Finally, we will show you a plan that includes the lowest amount of food recommended; if you eat less than this amount, you may suffer a loss of essential nutrients.

Are you ready? Get out your calculator and fill in the following information. Don't be intimidated by the math!

WEIGHT

Step 1: What is your weight in pounds? _____

    Carlos: ____187____

Step 2: Convert this to kilograms:

    Weight in pounds ÷ 2.2 = Weight in kilograms (kg.)

    _____ lb. ÷ 2.2 = _____ kg.

    Carlos: _187_ lb. ÷ 2.2 = _85_ kg.

Step 3: Plug the number you calculated in step 2 into the formula below. Use the correct formula for your gender.

    Women: 9.56 x kg. = FWeight*

        9.56 x _____ = _____

    Men: 13.75 x kg. = FWeight

        13.75 x _____ = _____

    Carlos: 13.75 x _85_ = _1168.75_

    Your FWeight: _____

    Carlos: FWeight: ____1168.75____

* *F* stands for "formula," as this is the number you will use in the formula to calculate your energy needs below.

HEIGHT

Step 1: What is your height in inches? _____

    Carlos: What is your height in inches? ___68 inches (5'8")___

Step 2: Convert this to centimeters:

Height in inches x 2.54 = Height in centimeters (cm.)

_____ in. x 2.54 = _____ cm.

Carlos: _____68_____ in. x 2.54 = _____172.72_____ cm.

Step 3: Plug the number you calculated in step 2 into the formula below. Use the correct formula for your gender.

Women: 1.85 x cm. = FHeight

1.85 x _____ = _____

Men: 5 x cm. = FHeight

5 x _____ = _____

Carlos: 5 x _172.72__ = _863.6__

Your FHeight: _____

Carlos: FHeight:____863.6___

AGE

Step 1: Your age in years: _____

Carlos: _39_____

Step 2: Plug your age into the formula below. Use the correct formula for your gender.

Women: 4.68 x age = FAge

4.68 x _____ = _____

Men: 6.76 x age = FAge

6.76 x _____ = _____

Carlos: 6.76 x _39_____ = _263.64__

Your FAge: _____

Carlos: FAge: ___263.64_____

ACTIVITY LEVEL

Step 1: Decide on your activity level.

Sedentary = You don't do any planned activity, such as working out at a gym. Also, the activity that's built into your daily life would not equal walking for about an hour a day if you put it all together. You work in an office where you sit most of the day, for example.

Active = You work out three to six times per week, getting your heart rate up for twenty to sixty minutes at a time. You might work out in a gym or you might get out and walk, bike, or swim. Or, the activity that's built into your daily life exceeds an hour per day of accumulated activity of an intensity no higher than that of a brisk walk.

Very active = You are training at the level of a competitive athlete (more than an hour per day). Or, your work is physically demanding or requires activity for numerous hours per day (for example, you are a mail carrier, mover, or manual laborer).

My current level of activity: _____

Carlos: _____*Sedentary*_____

Step 2: Choose the number that's right for you. This is your activity factor.

I live a sedentary lifestyle = 1.2

I live an active lifestyle = 1.4

I live a very active lifestyle = 1.6 to 2.0

My Activity Factor: _____

Carlos: _*1.2*_____

PUT IT ALL TOGETHER

Plug the numbers you calculated above into the formula below to determine your basal metabolic needs. The result is the amount of energy your body requires (from food) to stay alive. We will multiply this number by your activity factor to determine the energy your body needs to continue to live and be active. If you are currently sedentary, we encourage you to also calculate your energy needs as an active person, because you may decide to increase your physical activity as part of a healthy living or weight loss plan.

Women

655.1 + (FWeight) + (FHeight) – (FAge) = Basal Metabolic Needs

655.1 + _____ + _____ – _____ = _____

Now multiply your Basal Metabolic Needs by your Activity Factor:

Basal Metabolic Needs x Activity Factor = My Energy Needs

_____ x _____ = _____

If your activity level is sedentary, calculate your energy needs as they would be for an active person as well:

Basal Metabolic Needs x Activity Factor = My Energy Needs

_____ x __1.4__ = _____

Men:

66.47 + (FWeight) + (FHeight) − (FAge) = Basal Metabolic Needs

66.47 + _____ + _____ − _____ = _____

Carlos: 66.47 + _1168.75_ + __863.6__ − _263.64_ = _1835.18_

Now multiply your Basal Metabolic Needs by your Activity Factor:

Basal Metabolic Needs x Activity Factor = My Energy Needs

_____ x _____ = _____

Carlos: _1835.18_ x _1.2_ = _2202.216_

If your activity level is currently sedentary, calculate your energy needs as they would be for an active person as well:

Basal Metabolic Needs x Activity Factor = My Energy Needs

_____ x __1.4__ = _____

Carlos: _1835.18_ x __1.4__ = _2569.252_

Your Plan: How Much Can You Eat?

Before we develop your particular eating plan, we need to agree on what we will call a "serving" or a "portion." Many diet plans would have you weighing and measuring your food or buying prepackaged servings. But we want your eating to be as "normal" as possible, so we will base our servings or portions on those described in the American and Canadian Healthy Eating Guides, available online at www.my pyramid.gov and www.healthcanada.gc.ca/foodguide. The plan we will develop specifically for you, based on these portions, will be a healthy plan meant to work throughout your life.

FOOD GROUPS AND SERVING SIZES

Food guides separate foods into categories: grains, fruits and vegetables, dairy, and meat or meat alternatives. Fat is also considered separately, since it's an important nutrient in our diet. Each of the different "food groups" is made up of the basic building blocks we require to be healthy, or *macronutrients*: carbohydrates, protein, and fat. Carbohydrates and fat have both been thought of as unhealthy at various times, depending on the diet fad of the day. Most recently, dieters have been avoiding carbohydrates; earlier, dieters were trying to live a "fat-free" life. However, it's important to understand that all of these macronutrients are essential for good health. None of them magically makes you fat, nor will avoiding them automatically make you thinner. In fact, research is clear that the composition of weight-loss diets—the proportion of protein, carbohydrate, or fat—is not what works to achieve weight loss; it's reducing calories that matters (Melanson and Dwyer 2002). But good health depends on your taking in an appropriate balance of these macronutrients.

In order to have good health, we also need to have the right vitamins and minerals in our diet. These are called *micronutrients*. Many health food stores and companies make and sell nutritional supplements, and their advertisements might lead you to believe that you don't actually need to eat food to get the micronutrients you need. However, your body was designed to consume vitamins and minerals from whole foods, and micronutrients in supplements have sometimes been found to cause harm while micronutrients found in food almost never do (Food and Nutrition Board, National Research Council 1989). One of the reasons nutritionists separate foods into different food groups is that each food group is particularly strong in certain micronutrients. If you miss out on certain food groups, you miss out on particular micronutrients that are essential for good health.

In the table below, we give you examples of foods in each food group and describe serving sizes.

Examples and Serving Sizes*	
Grains:	
1 piece of bread, small tortilla, small muffin, small dinner roll 1 pancake or waffle ½ of a pita, bagel, English muffin, large tortilla, kaiser roll, hamburger or hot dog bun ½ c. rice, potato,** pasta, couscous 3 c. popcorn 1 granola bar	
Fruits	**Vegetables**
1 whole fruit: apple, banana, peach, pear, or other fruit ½ c. berries or cut fruit ½ c. juice	Broccoli spear, whole carrot, or equivalent 1 c. of leafy vegetables (such as lettuce) ½ c. of vegetables or juice
Dairy	
1 c. milk (cow or soy) ¾ c. yogurt 2 cheese sticks, 1.5 oz. cheese, or 2 sandwich-size slices of cheese	

Meat and Fish	Meat Alternatives
1 piece of steak, chicken, or pork, the size of a deck of cards	¾ c. beans or lentils
1 piece of fish, the size of your palm and fingers	Soy meat alternative (as indicated on package)
2 or 3 fish sticks or chicken strips	2 tbs. peanut butter
2.5 oz. luncheon meat or tuna	¼ c. hummus

*   *Note:* When reviewing the above table, please remember that for some foods, it would be acceptable to have two or three servings at one sitting. For example, a sandwich for lunch would be two servings of grains (two slices of bread).

**   We know potatoes are vegetables, but they are often the "starchy" part of a meal, so we will count them as grains.)

SO WHAT SPECIFICALLY ARE YOUR RECOMMENDED SERVINGS PER DAY?

Now that you have calculated your daily energy needs and you have a good idea of the typical serving sizes, we can take a look at what you will eat in a day.

Healthy Living Plan. Round your energy needs to the nearest hundred (for example, if your energy needs are 2,156 calories, you can round up to 2,200). Write this estimate of your energy needs in the space just above the chart below. If your number falls between two of the numbers on the chart, add or subtract food servings from the nearest number's column according to your preference. For example, if you are at 2,400 calories, you might choose to drop a dairy serving from the 2,500 column, rather than drop a grain or fruit-and-vegetable serving. (Note that it's the grains, fruits and vegetables, and dairy servings that increase from 2,200 to 2,500, so these would be the groups you would choose from.)

Weight-Loss Plan (Balanced Deficit Plan): Start by rounding your energy needs to the nearest hundred (for example, if your calorie needs are 2,156, you can round up to 2,200). Because you are planning to lose weight, you will subtract 500 calories from this total. For example, if you have estimated your energy needs to be 2,200, your weight loss plan will be 2,200 − 500 = 1,700. If your number falls between or below two of the numbers on the chart, you will add or subtract food servings according to your preference to meet your energy needs. For example, to achieve the goal of taking in 1,700 calories, you might choose to eliminate a grain from the 1,800 column. Your servings would be six grains, six fruits or vegetables, three dairy foods, two meats, and five fats. The minimum number of servings we would ever recommend without close medical supervision are the following: five grains, five fruits and vegetables, two dairy foods, two meats, and three fats. We give a sample of this plan below.

What About Calories? We would prefer that you think about your food in terms of food groups and servings, and forget about calories. However, we do make the assumption that you are not consistently picking the *richest* choices (for example, muffins and granola for grains) or the *lightest* choices (for example, celery and cucumbers for vegetables). Instead, we want you to aim for the middle by balancing rich and light choices. If you would like to check your choices, you can measure them against the following general standards for individual food group servings: a serving of grains averages 100 calories, fruits 75 calories, vegetables 25 calories, dairy 100 calories, meat and meat alternatives 150 calories; and fats 50 to 70 calories.

My energy needs (rounded to nearest hundred): _____

Calories	1,800	2,000	2,200	2,500	2,700	3,000	3,200	3,500
Grains	7	7	8	9	10	11	11	12
Fruits and vegetables*	6	7	7	8	9	10	11	12
Dairy	3	3	3	4	4	4	5	5
Meats and meat alternatives	2	2.5	3	3	3	3	3.5	4
Extra fat servings	5	6	6	6	7	9	9	10

* *Note:* Try to make sure that you choose equally from fruits and from vegetables.

Write out your food group servings here:

Grains: _____

Fruits and vegetables: _____

Dairy: _____

Meats and meat alternatives: _____

Fats: _____

Carlos's weight falls in the overweight range and his waist circumference suggests that he's at higher risk for health problems. Weight loss is an option for Carlos. However, Carlos made the decision to try healthy living first, since he greatly enjoys food and can't imagine following a restrictive eating plan. He hopes that, by improving his eating and increasing his physical activity, he will see improvements to his health.

Carlos decided to work on a plan based on his current activity level (sedentary), knowing that he would change the plan once he became regularly active. Carlos rounded his energy needs down to 2,200 (from 2,202.216) and his food group servings are listed below:

7   *Grains*

7   *Fruits and vegetables*

3   *Dairy*

3   *Meats or meat alternatives*

6   *Fats*

What About Fat Servings? The previous food serving chart was developed to give you the optimum balance of food groups (and macronutrients), as well as a heart-healthy, low-fat diet. This means that between 25 and 30 percent of your overall calories, or energy, will come from fat if you follow this plan. Half of the fat is assumed to be inherent in your food. For example, both dairy and meat or meat alternative products are assumed to have fat built in. As is consistent with food guides around the world, we encourage you to make low-fat choices when you can, such as skim milk, milk with 1 or 2 percent fat, or lean meats. The second half of the fat in your diet is "added" fat. In other words, fat that you add to your food or "treats" you enjoy as part of your diet. The previous chart assumes that a single fat serving is equal to 5 grams of fat. Almost all food is labeled in a way that provides the number of grams of fat in a serving. If, for example, a treat you choose has 11 grams of fat on the nutrition label, we would estimate that to be about 2 fat servings according to the chart. As is the case with the other food groups, we don't assume you will only have one fat serving at a time; most desserts, for example, would be two or three servings. Take a look at the following table to see how to count fat servings:

Examples of Fat Servings (Equal to 5 Grams of Fat)

Served on or with food:

⅛ avocado

1 teaspoon butter, margarine, or oil

1 tablespoon cream cheese

2 tablespoons heavy cream (10 percent fat)

2 tablespoons gravy

10 green olives

8 black olives

2 teaspoons salad dressing (regular)

2 tablespoons light or low-fat salad dressing

2 tablespoons sour cream

½ tablespoon regular mayonnaise, or 1 tablespoon light mayonnaise

"Decadent" treats:

⅓ chocolate bar (60 g.)

⅓ package candy-coated chocolate pieces (60 g.)

⅓ bag potato chips (55 g.)

1 or 2 chocolate chip cookies (30 g.)

¼ cup ice cream (regular)

½ danish or doughnut

½ piece chocolate cake

⅓ piece pie

2 Rice Krispies squares

2 doughnut holes

Healthy fat alternatives*

1 tablespoon (15 ml.) almonds, pecans (3-5 individual nuts)

4 teaspoons (20 ml.) cashews, pistachios (6 cashews, 10-12 pistachios)

4 teaspoons (20 ml.) pumpkin seeds

1 tablespoon (15 ml.) sunflower seeds

2 teaspoons (10 ml.) peanut butter

1-by-1-inch piece (15 g.) cheese

* Please note that these nut and seed amounts are not those used when substituting for meat. These are nut and seed servings to be used as "extra" fats.

Restaurant eating:

For deep-fried foods (such as fries) assume 3 fats.

For pan-fried foods (such as hamburger) assume 2 fats.

For sautéed foods (such as broccoli sautéed in olive oil) assume 2 fats.

For stir-fried foods (such as Chinese food) assume 2 fats.

Condiments, Garnishes (or Toppings), Alcohol, and Candy

Condiments (syrup, jam, and so on): Condiments that you add to food don't need to be counted, as long as you use them in reasonable amounts.

Vegetable toppings and garnishes (a lettuce leaf on a sandwich, pickle slices, and so on): Unless you really think that the amount would equal a complete serving, don't count these toppings.

Alcohol: Alcoholic drinks contain calories and need to be considered as part of your intake. But of more concern is the role that alcohol plays in increasing appetite and therefore food intake (Melanson and Dwyer 2002). If you have chosen a weight-loss plan, we recommend that you avoid alcohol. If you are following the healthy living plan, we recommend that you not exceed the recommendation of one drink per day for women, and two drinks per day for men (see International Center for Alcohol Policies [ICAP] website [2007] for international guidelines for alcohol intake). If your alcohol intake is more the exception than the rule—in other words, you rarely drink alcoholic beverages—then you need not count it as part of your meal plan. If you drink alcohol more than twice per week, then we would suggest that you allocate two fat servings per drink toward this.

Candy: In general, one serving as listed on the package (between 100 and 120 calories) will count as two of your fat servings. Do not use up more than three of your fat servings on candy, since you need fat as a healthy part of your diet. Fat also gives you better satiety than sugar does, keeping you from feeling hungry.

How to Plan Your Actual Day

You have figured out your energy needs and know how many servings of the various food groups you need, but how do you plan a real day? First we will give you the guidelines for planning a day, and then we will take you through the steps to plan your food intake. We will use Carlos's plan as an example of a "healthy living day" and Janice's plan as an example of a "weight loss" day, and then we will provide you with an example of a low-calorie diet (the lowest you should go without medical monitoring).

Guidelines for Healthy Eating

1. Each meal has a minimum of three food groups. Larger meals usually have four.

2. Eat your first meal within an hour of waking up and make sure your meals are no longer than three to four hours apart until you go to sleep.

3. Snacks should be made up of food groups you are weak in (food groups you have trouble getting enough of, such as fruits, vegetables, and dairy) and usually include two food groups.

4. To improve satiety and keep you from getting hungry too quickly, make sure your snacks and meals include a combination of carbohydrates (fruits, vegetables, and grains) and fats or protein (dairy, meats and meat alternatives, treat foods).

5. Choose low-fat foods, *not* foods that are either high in fat or have no fat.

6. Add a modest amount of fat to your food throughout the day, have one decadent treat a day, or both.

Creating Your Eating Plan

Next, you will take your energy requirements and design a plan based on the number of servings recommended for you.

To plan your day, follow the steps below to fill in the "Planning Chart":

Step 1: Write in the times you wake up and eat your meals.

Step 2: Put in snack times wherever you'll have more than four hours between meals or between a meal and bedtime.

Step 3: Start with grains and divide them up between meals. If your total number of grains allows, have two per meal. If you have grains left, add a serving of grains to one of your snack times.

Step 4: Repeat step 3 for each of the remaining food groups. Try to divide them evenly throughout your day.

Step 5: Consider where you will add fats to your meals. If you like "dressing up" your food (adding butter, dressing, gravy, and the like), you will want your fat servings at your meals. If you need a treat, then make sure to save some of your fats (two or three is common) for your treat; pick a time of day when eating your treat will be completely satisfying (not on the run or while working, for example) and try to have your treat at a time when you have already eaten a meal or snack so you aren't too hungry.

Step 6: Create sample meals to match your food groups.

PLANNING CHART

Knowing the food group servings you are aiming for in a given meal allows you to be quite flexible in planning your food intake. You may want to take a look at Carlos's and Janice's plans to help you fill in your own chart.

Time	Food Groups	Meal 1	Meal 2	Meal 3
Wake: _____ a.m.				
Breakfast: _____ a.m.	Grains: _____			
	Fruits or veggies: _____			
	Dairy: _____			
	Meat or alternative: ____			
	Fats: _____			
Snack: _____ a.m.				
Lunch: _____ a.m. or p.m.	Grains: _____			
	Fruits or veggies: _____			
	Dairy: _____			
	Meat or alternative: ____			
	Fats: _____			
Snack: _____ p.m.				
Dinner: _____ p.m.	Grains: _____			
	Fruits or veggies: _____			
	Dairy: _____			
	Meat or alternative: ____			
	Fats: _____			
Snack: _____ p.m.				
Bed: _____ p.m..				

HEALTHY LIVING: CARLOS'S PLAN

Time	Food Groups	Meal 1	Meal 2	Meal 3
Wake: 6:30 a.m.				
Breakfast: 7:30 a.m.	Grains: __2__	2 pc. toast	2 servings dry cereal	2 pancakes
	Fruits or veggies: __1__	1/2 c. OJ	1 banana	1/2 c. berries
	Dairy: __1__	3/4 c. yogurt	1 c. milk	3/4 c. yogurt
	Meat or alternative: __1__	2 poached eggs	2 scrambled eggs	2 small sausages
	Fats: __1__	1 tsp. marg.	1 tsp. marg.	1 tsp. marg.
Snack: 10:00 a.m.	1 Fruit or veggie	1 pc. fruit	1 pc. fruit	1 pc. fruit
	1 Grain	1 granola bar	1 granola bar	1 granola bar
Lunch: 12:00 noon	Grains: __2__	2 pc. bread or 1 bun	1 large tortilla	1 c. pasta
	Fruits or veggies: __2__	1/2 c. baby carrots and 1 apple (and lettuce and tomato on a sandwich)	1 c. lettuce, 1/2 c. chopped tomato	1 c. chopped veggies (green pepper, tomato)
	Dairy: __1__	1 c. choc. milk	1.5 oz. grated cheese	3 oz. feta cheese
	Meat or alternative: __1__	75 g. cold cuts	sautéed chicken	3/4 c. chickpeas
	Fats: __1__	1 tbs. low-fat mayo, mustard	1 tsp. marg. to sauté chicken	Low-fat Greek salad dressing (5 g. fat)
Snack: 3:30 p.m.	1 Dairy	3/4 c. yogurt	3/4 c. yogurt	3/4 c. yogurt
	1 Fruit or veggie	1 pc. fruit	1 pc. fruit	1 pc. fruit
Dinner: 6:00 p.m.	Grains: __2__	1 c. rice	1 medium potato	1 c. pasta
	Fruits or veggies: __2__	1 c. sauteed veggies	2 spears broccoli	1/2 c. tomato sauce and 1 c. lettuce
	Dairy: __0__			
	Meat or alternative: __1__	Steak	Roast chicken	75 g. hamburger for meat sauce
	Fats: __2__	2 tsp. oil	4 tbs. sour cream	4 tsp. regular salad dressing
Snack: 8:00 p.m.	1 grain	3 c. popcorn	3 c. popcorn	3 c. popcorn
	1 fat	1 tsp. butter	1 tbs. butter	1 tsp. butter
Bed: 10:30 p.m.				

WEIGHT LOSS: JANICE'S PLAN

Janice's weight falls in the obese range, and she's quite concerned about her health risks because of her father's recent heart attack. She's an organized and determined person in many ways, so she decided she would try the weight-loss plan. Janice's energy needs were based on an active lifestyle and were calculated to be 2,301.31, which she rounded down to 2,300. Her weight-loss plan totals 500 calories fewer than her energy needs (in other words, 2,300 − 500 = 1,800).

Her food servings for an 1,800-calorie plan are as follows:

7   grains

6   fruits and vegetables

3   dairy

2   meats or meat alternatives

5   fats

PLANNING CHART

Below is a sample plan created for Janice:

Time	Food Groups	Meal 1	Meal 2	Meal 3
Wake: 7:00 a.m.				
Breakfast: 8:00 a.m.	Grains: ___2___	2 servings dry cereal	2 servings oatmeal	1 English muffin
	Fruits or veggies: ___1___	Banana	1/2 c. berries	1 tomato
	Dairy: ___1___	1 c. milk	1 c. milk (oatmeal cooked in milk)	1.5 oz. cheese melted on English muffin
	Meat or alternative: ___0___			
	Fats: ___0___			
Snack: none				
Lunch: 12:00 noon	Grains: ___2___	2 pc. toast	1 small bagel	1 bun
	Fruits or veggies: ___1___	1/2 c. baby carrots and 1 apple	Veggie soup and apple	1/2 c. baby carrots and 1 tomato
	Dairy: ___1___	3/4 cup yogurt	3/4 c. yogurt	3/4 c. yogurt
	Meat or alternative: ___1___	2 tbs. peanut butter	75 g. luncheon meat	75 g. tuna
	Fats: ___0–1___		1 tbs. low-fat mayo	1 tbs. low-fat mayo

Snack: 3:30 p.m.	1 Grain	Dry cereal	Crackers	Granola bar
	1 Dairy	1 c. milk	1.5 oz. cheese	3/4 c. yogurt
	1 Fruit	1/2 c. berries	Apple	Pear
Dinner: 6:00 p.m.	Grains: __2__	1 cup rice	1 medium potato	1 medium potato
	Fruits or veggies: __2__	1 c. stir-fry veggies	1/2 c. green beans, 1/2 c. corn	1 c. lettuce, 1/2 c. chopped veggies
	Dairy: __0__			
	Meat or alternative: __1__	Chicken	Steak	Salmon
	Fats: __2__	2 tsp. oil	2 tsp. marg.	2 tbs. light salad dressing, 1 tsp. marg.
Snack: 8:00 p.m.	Treat (2 to 3 fats)	55 g. bag potato chips	Frozen yogurt	1 large cookie (10 g. fat)
Bed: 11:00 p.m.				

LOW-CALORIE WEIGHT LOSS PLAN: DON'T GO LOWER THAN THIS!

This plan is based on the minimum servings required to meet your nutritional needs. If you choose to follow this plan and you find yourself too hungry, or if you have lost between 5 and 15 percent of your original body weight, you should return to the balanced deficit weight-loss plan described previously (your body's energy needs minus 500 calories). The following low-calorie weight loss plan allows you to eat five grains, five fruits and vegetables, two dairy items, two meats, and three added fat servings.

Planning Chart

Following is a sample low-calorie weight loss plan:

Time	Food Groups	Meal 1	Meal 2	Meal 3
Wake: *7:00 am*				
Breakfast: *8:00 a.m.*	Grains: __1__	1 serving dry cereal	1 serving oatmeal	1/2 English muffin
	Fruits or veggies: __1__	Banana	1/2 c. berries	1 tomato
	Dairy: __1__	1 c. milk	1 c. milk (oatmeal cooked in milk)	1.5 oz. cheese melted on English muffin
	Meat or alternative: __0__			
	Fats: __0__			
Snack: *none*				
Lunch: *12:00 noon*	Grains: __2__	2 pc. toast	1 small bagel	1 bun
	Fruits or veggies: __1__	1 apple	Veggie soup	1/2 c. baby carrots
	Dairy: __1__	3/4 c. yogurt	3/4 c. yogurt	3/4 c. yogurt
	Meat or alternative: __1__	2 tbs. peanut butter	75 g. luncheon meat	75 g. tuna
	Fats: __1__	2 small cookies	1 tbs. Low-fat mayo	1 tbs. low-fat mayo
Snack: *3:30 p.m.*	1 Fruit	1/2 c. berries	Apple	Pear
Dinner: *6:00 p.m.*	Grains: __2__	1 c. rice	1 medium potato	1 medium potato
	Fruits or veggies: __2__	1 c. stir-fry veggies	1/2 c. green beans, 1/2 c. corn	1 c. lettuce, 1/2 c. chopped veggies
	Dairy: __0__			
	Meat or alternative: __1__	Chicken	Steak	Salmon
	Fats: __2__	2 tsp. oil	2 tsp. marg.	2 tbs. light salad dressing, 1 tsp. marg.
Snack: *none*				
Bed: *11:00 p.m.*				

PUTTING THE PLAN INTO ACTION: TIPS FOR SUCCESS

You have your plan, and you know your nutritional needs and health goals. Before you begin, read the tips below to help improve your chances of success.

Jump In or Make Gradual Change?

It may seem obvious that you should jump right in, now that you have come up with your plan. If you can do this, go right ahead. The reality is that, for some people, changing an entire day or week may just seem too overwhelming. If this is the case, we recommend changing your eating habits more gradually, focusing on one meal or snack per week. Start by changing your breakfast every day the first week; then focus on another meal or snack the next week, and so on. Each week, improve a new meal or snack until you are following your complete plan. Don't worry if this seems like a slow process. Remember that you are making changes that are supposed to last you a lifetime. There's no need to hurry. The important thing is to get there.

SHOPPING

To put your plan into action, you are going to need the food that's on your plan. We encouraged you to plan for three different options per meal. Feel free to expand on this and plan for every day of the week, especially dinner, since this tends to be the meal with the most variety. Or, you can just repeat each meal once (two repetitions of three different meals) and assume you might go out for the seventh meal. Whatever you decide, sit down with your plan and create a grocery list. Organize your list with the same food group headings you use in your plan: "Grains," "Fruits and veggies," "Dairy," "Meats and meat alternatives," and "Added fats." Bring the list with you and buy *only* the things you have written down. If you are feeding a family, buy breakfast, lunch, and snack food for yourself, and adjust the amounts to meet your family's needs for the meals you eat together. Create a separate list for your family's meal needs, especially for the meals that you do not eat together. It's important to try to limit the quantity of foods that you feel less in control around. Plan carefully to avoid preparing more food than you or your family needs; if you really have difficulty with treat foods, you may want to choose something you can buy in single-serving packages.

TOO MUCH OR TOO LITTLE CHOICE?

The eating plan we have given you is intended to provide a wide range of choice for how you meet your serving requirements. However, too much choice can sometimes lead to a loss of control and overeating. Planning your food intake and sticking to your plan can help you have the best of both worlds; you can plan variety but limit choice by following your plan. If you find that even this amount of choice puts you at risk of overeating, we suggest that you limit breakfast, lunch, and snacks to the same choices every day and allow yourself variety at dinner. We strongly recommend that you work hard to follow your plan to the letter—both in the timing and the food choices. We call this *mechanical* eating. You don't have to think about what you are doing; just follow your plan. Eating *mechanically* will help you to develop and maintain good habits. If you are used to eating in response to emotional triggers, you will find that mechanical eating helps you to separate the food from your feelings. We will help you to find different ways to manage your emotions in chapter 8.

SHIFT WORK

If you work evening or overnight shifts, you may be wondering how to plan your eating. Our "Guidelines for Healthy Eating" (earlier in this chapter) recommend that you start eating within an hour of waking and continue eating every three to four hours until you go to bed. The same rule applies whether you wake at 7:00 a.m. or at 4:00 p.m. The main difference might be the choice of food. Let's consider what you might eat if you wake at 4:00 p.m. If you prefer to match what your family members are eating, you might start with a small snack and join your family for supper at 6:00 p.m. You might have a snack at 10:00 p.m. and "lunch" at midnight. You might have another snack at 3:00 p.m. and a small "breakfast" at 7:00 a.m. before you go to bed for the day.

TIME TO START: PLANNING AND EVALUATING YOUR PROGRESS

We have designed a daily planning sheet for you to set up your week and evaluate how you are meeting your goals. Feel free to photocopy the blank sheet and use it for every day of the week. On the sheet is a place for you to plan and track your food and the servings you eat. You are also asked to state your goal for the day. You may start your healthy-living or weight-loss plan by trying to regularly eat one meal, one snack, or all your meals, or even meet your entire plan; the choice of how to begin is yours. But whatever you choose, *be specific*. Once you have defined your goal, put all your heart into meeting that goal. If you feel overwhelmed, scale back and set a less ambitious goal, and gradually work from there. You also have a space to record what you think got in the way of your goal. This is meant to get you started thinking and will help later as we troubleshoot obstacles. Chapters 7 through 9 will help you look at these obstacles and work to overcome them.

My Daily Plan and How I Am Doing

What I plan to eat today: (Fill in times, food choices, and amounts.)	Food Servings*					What I actually ate: (Fill in times, food choices, and amounts.)	Food Servings*				
	G	F & V	D	M & A	F & O		G	F & V	D	M & A	F & O
Wake up: Breakfast:						Wake up: Breakfast:					
Snack:						Snack:					
Lunch:						Lunch:					
Snack:						Snack:					
Dinner:						Dinner:					
Snack:						Snack:					
Total Servings:						**Total Servings:**					

What my goal was today (for example, follow plan at breakfast, do all meals according to plan, or do all meals and snacks):

What got in the way of achieving my goal (for example, circumstance, emotions, people, or other things):

* G = Grains, F & V = Fruits and veggies, D = Dairy, M & A = Meat and meat alternatives, F = Fats

CHAPTER CHECKLIST

You have completed this chapter when:

○ You have estimated your energy needs.

○ You have written out your food servings.

○ You have planned three sample days using the Planning Chart.

○ You have set a goal for changing your eating.

○ You have used the "My Daily Plan" sheet to plan out your week, set your goals, and record any obstacles.

What do you do next and when?

○ Move on at any time to chapter 6 and plan your activity.

○ Use the "My Daily Plan" sheet each day for the next week and record your eating.

○ Don't be discouraged if you are having difficulty meeting your food goals in this first week. It's okay if you run into problems, because that's what you will be dealing with next. After one week of recording on your "My Daily Plan" sheet, begin reading chapters 7 through 9. These chapters are intended to help you overcome any obstacles you are facing in your attempts to meet your eating and activity goals.

You are ready to eat—enjoy!

CHAPTER 6

Changing Your Lifestyle: Designing Your Activity Plan

Is physical activity a challenge for you? Many people know it's good for them and know they should be doing more but just can't seem to make happen. Whatever your feelings about physical activity, it's a change that will probably have the greatest positive impact on both your physical and mental health. The good news is that there's a physical activity plan that will work for just about everyone—including you.

WHY BOTHER TO BE ACTIVE?

You are looking to manage your weight most likely because of health concerns or because of body dissatisfaction. So let's look at the role that physical activity plays in each of these areas.

Physical Activity and Health

Some researchers believe that physical fitness is far more important in reducing health risks than achieving a particular body weight. Physical activity has been shown to reduce the risk of diseases such as heart disease, diabetes, and cancer (Warburton, Nicol, and Bredin 2006). It also has short-term benefits, such as improved functioning of your immune system (Gleeson 2007).

So, let's get specific. Take a look at the following list of health benefits associated with physical activity, and make a check mark next to those that are of value to you.

Physical Health Benefits of Fitness Checklist

☐ Prevention of heart disease

☐ Prevention of diabetes

☐ Prevention of cancer

☐ Prevention of osteoporosis

☐ Strengthening of your immune system

☐ Prevention of injury, due to better balance, improved coordination, and stronger and more flexible muscles

☐ Prevention of back pain

☐ Relief from constipation

☐ Relief from chronic joint pain

☐ Relief from insomnia

☐ Stable weight over your lifetime or to help maintain weight loss

Physical Activity and Mental Health (and Body Satisfaction)

If you see physical activity as a way to significantly increase your rate of weight loss, you are bound to be disappointed. Physical activity has not been found to result in weight loss beyond what you can achieve from reducing food intake (Foreyt et al. 1993). However, physical activity can benefit your mental health in general, and your satisfaction with your body in particular. In fact, one of the most exciting and growing bodies of research is the study of the impact of physical activity on mental health (Stathopoulou et al. 2006). Physical activity was found to significantly reduce depressed mood and anxiety (particularly panic disorder), reduce cravings and increase abstinence rates in alcoholism, and reduce binge eating in people suffering from eating disorders (both bulimia and binge-eating disorder).

Mental Health Benefits of Fitness Checklist

Take a look at the following mental health benefits and make a check mark next to those that are of value to you.

☐ Reduction of binge eating

☐ Stress relief

☐ Increased alertness

☐ Increased energy

☐ Improved mood

☐ Lowered anxiety

☐ Reduction in cravings for alcohol

☐ Improved body image

☐ Increased sex drive

Why Should You Bother?

Take a look at the physical and mental health benefits of being physically active that you checked off on the previous list. Write the ones that seem most important to you on the lines below. Can you think of any that aren't in the list?

My Personal Reasons to Improve My Fitness Level

_____

_____

_____

_____

Now that you have recorded your reasons for wanting to increase your physical activity, we will describe the components of physical activity and ask you to rate your current level of physical activity. We will help you identify the types of activity that you will enjoy or at least find easy to fit into your life, even if you still have doubts that you can do it.

Janice had dabbled in activity but had had difficulty maintaining anything she started because of her travel. She was determined to come up with a plan that would work with her schedule. Her concern about the health of her heart was her biggest motivation.

WHAT EXACTLY DO WE MEAN BY "PHYSICAL ACTIVITY"?

There are three types of physical activity that significantly improve fitness:

Cardiovascular ("Cardio") or Aerobic Activities

Cardio activities include those in which your whole body moves continuously, often in a rhythmic manner, over a long period. Examples of cardio activities are brisk walking, jogging, running, swimming, and biking. Ideally, you will engage in some kind of cardio activity three to six times a week, giving your-self a day off to allow your muscles to recover. On any single day, you don't need to do the activity all in one go (for example, walking for sixty minutes straight), but it's recommended that you accumulate activity in at least ten-minute chunks of time. For example, you may walk ten minutes to the bus stop in the morning, go on a twenty-minute walk at lunch, walk ten minutes from the bus stop home after work, and walk the dog for twenty minutes when you get home in the evening. The total daily time recommended for cardio activities ranges from twenty to sixty minutes. The more intense the activity, the less time you need to be active. Almost all the physical and mental health benefits have been found for people who are active four to five days per week, at moderate to high intensity.

Muscular Strength or Resistance Activities

Strength training includes any activity that requires pushing or pulling with effort, either with machines or free weights, or in the form of exercises using your own body weight, such as push-ups, squats, and sit-ups. Strength training can be built into your daily life through such things as yard work, carrying children or groceries, scrubbing tubs, or vacuuming carpets.

If you are looking for a significant increase in muscle size, you have to push, pull, and lift weights so heavy that you can't maintain good form (or posture) after eight to twelve repetitions. You will likely need a personal trainer to make sure that you are balancing the muscle groups correctly and maintaining good form. If you are aiming for toned but not bulky muscles, you will choose lighter loads and do more repetitions, although not more than twelve to twenty times in one go (or "set"). Whether you are looking for larger muscles or good muscle tone, you would never repeat each set of repetitions more than two or three times. Because your muscles need time to heal and become stronger after these sessions, you should never do strength training with the same body parts two days in a row. Cardio and strength activities have been shown to have equal benefits to physical and mental health. As is the case with cardio activities, the greatest benefits have been found in people who engage in this form of exercise four days a week, at moderate to high intensity.

Flexibility Training

Flexibility training includes activities where the muscles are being gently stretched. Stretching and increasing flexibility can be an important part of preventing injury. Muscles are most safely and effectively stretched when they have been warmed up, so it's recommended that you spend at least a few minutes moving around before you try to stretch your muscles.

To prevent injury and stiffness, it's important to lengthen your muscles by stretching after exercising, while the muscles are still warm. Once you get in the habit of stretching, you will look forward to the pleasure of releasing those muscles.

As long as you are warmed up, you can stretch your muscles every day of the week. Never bounce when stretching, because this can injure the muscle. Instead, you should gradually stretch the muscle until you feel mild tension but not pain, and hold your stretch for a minimum of twenty to thirty seconds, and a maximum of sixty seconds; this type of stretching is called "static" stretching. A number of physical activities have stretching built into them, such as dancing, curling, yoga, bowling, golfing, and gardening; these involve "dynamic" stretching. You may need help learning how to stretch your muscles, and a personal trainer, videos, or books can be very useful in teaching you the proper technique.

HOW DO YOU KNOW IF YOUR ACTIVITY IS "INTENSE" ENOUGH?

If you are going to experience benefits to your physical and mental health, the intensity of your activity will need to fall within a recommended range. For cardio activities, intensity is measured according to your increased or "working" heart rate (HR). Follow the four steps below to calculate your "working" heart-rate range.

Step 1

Take your pulse for sixty seconds in the morning after waking up naturally (the sound of an alarm clock causes your body to release adrenaline and speed up your heart rate) or after a period of rest, when you feel relaxed and haven't consumed any caffeine or stimulants. To take your pulse, try placing your finger on the side of your neck or below your thumb on your wrist.

Write your resting HR here: _____

Step 2

Write your age and resting heart rate in the spaces in the formula below. You will need a calculator. Enter the numbers and perform the numerical operations one after the other to arrive at your minimum working heart rate.

220 -_____ - _____ x 0.65 = _____ ÷ 6 = _____
      (your age)   (resting HR)   (60 seconds)   (10 seconds)

Write your 60-second minimum here: _____

Write your 10-second minimum here: _____

Step 3

Next, enter your age and resting heart rate and calculate your maximum working heart rate below.

220 -_____ - _____ x 0.85 = _____ ÷ 6 = _____
      (your age)   (resting HR)   (60 seconds)   (10 seconds)

Write your 60-second maximum here: _____

Write your 10-second maximum here: _____

Your Working Heart Rate Zone

When you are exercising and your ten-second heart rate falls between the minimum and maximum you calculated above, you are in your "working heart rate zone." If your heart rate falls close to the minimum, you are exercising at a moderate intensity, which would be appropriate for longer sessions. If your heart rate rises closer to the maximum, you are working at a high intensity, which would be appropriate for shorter sessions.

A less technical way of estimating intensity is called the "talk test." If you can easily hold a conversation while exercising, your level of activity is probably in the low-intensity range. If you can manage two- or three-word phrases, you are likely working in the moderate- to high-intensity range. If you can't manage even two- or three-word phrases, your level of intensity is too high.

EVALUATE YOUR OWN LEVEL OF PHYSICAL ACTIVITY

Now that you understand the different components and intensity levels of physical activity, you can evaluate your current level of activity.

Your Cardio Level

Answer the questions below to determine your cardio activity level.

Frequency. Over a typical seven-day period, how many times do you engage in cardio activity that's long and intense enough to cause an increase in your heart rate?

- ☐ Rarely or never   You are sedentary.

- ☐ Once or twice   Pretty good—you're close to where you should be.

- ☐ Between 3 and 6 times   Excellent! This will leave you fit.

- ☐ Every day   This is good, but you need a day of rest

- ☐ Twice a day or more   You are exercising too much for your health and joints.

Duration. When you engage in cardio activity, how long do you typically exercise in each session?

- ☐ Less than 10 minutes   Try for 10-minute chunks.

- ☐ 10 minutes, once   You're close—just add one more 10-minute chunk per day!

- ☐ 10-minute chunks,   Excellent—this is a manageable approach. 2 to 6 times

- ☐ 20 to 60 minutes,   Excellent—this is a good workout. continuously

- ☐ More than 60 minutes   This quantity of exercising is hard on your body.

Intensity. When you engage in cardio activity, how hard do you feel you are working?

☐ I am making a light effort.   You might need to work a little harder.

☐ I am making a moderate   This is an excellent level for a duration of 30 to 60 minutes
effort.

☐ I am making an intense   This is an excellent level for a duration of 20 to 30 minutes.
effort.

What changes would you need to make in order to bring your cardio activity into healthy guidelines (20-60 minutes, 3-6 times per week)?

Your Muscular Strength or Resistance Level

Frequency. Over a typical seven-day period, how many times do you engage in muscular work requiring pushing, pulling, lifting, and the like?

☐ Never   Muscles will be weak and out of condition.

☐ Once a week   A good start—can you add one more?

☐ 2 to 4 times a week   Excellent—make sure to skip a day between workouts.

☐ 4 to 7 times a week   Your muscles need a day to recover between workouts.

☐ 2 sessions a day, every day   This is counterproductive—too much!

Intensity. How many times can you repeat the activity *before tiring or losing your form*?

Number of Repetitions	For Greater Strength	For Greater Endurance
☐ Less than 8 repetitions	Your weights are too heavy, or the activity you are choosing is too hard.	
☐ 8 to 12 repetitions	This is just right to increase strength.	Your weights are too heavy; this level of intensity is better for building strength.
☐ 12 to 20 repetitions	This level of intensity and repetition is too light for building strength.	This is perfect for building endurance.
☐ More than 20 repetitions		This is too many repetitions; you are at risk of developing a repetitive injury.

Duration. How many times do you repeat a set of repetitions?

☐ 1 set of repetitions   A good start—can you add one more?

☐ 2 to 3 sets of repetitions   This is effective for building strength.

☐ 2 to 4 sets of repetitions   This is effective for building endurance.

☐ More than 3 or 4 sets   You are doing too many sets and may be at risk of injury.

What changes would *you* need to make for your strength training activity to fall within healthy guidelines (2-3 set of 12-20 repetitions, 3 to 4 times per week)?

_____

Your Flexibility Level

Frequency. Over a typical seven-day period, how frequently do you engage in stretching?

☐ Never   You are at risk of injury.

☐ 1 or 2 times   Try to stretch more consistently.

☐ 3 to 6 times   Good—you are likely stretching after each workout.

☐ Every day   Good—make sure to warm up before you stretch.

Duration. Each time you stretch a muscle, how long do you hold the stretch?

☐ Less than 20 seconds   This is not enough time to properly stretch.

☐ 20 to 30 seconds   This is a bit on the short side, but it's acceptable.

☐ 30 to 60 seconds   This is an ideal length of time to hold a stretch.

☐ More than 60 seconds   Your stretching time is longer than necessary.

Intensity. Each time you stretch, you push yourself until:

☐ You feel mild tension   Just right!

☐ You feel pain   Too far! You risk injury.

What changes would *you* need to make for your flexibility level to fall within healthy guidelines (3-6 times per week holding each stretch for 30-60 seconds)?

_____

HOW COULD YOU IMPROVE YOUR FITNESS?

Now that you have assessed your fitness level, you can identify areas for improvement. We will help you plan for change, but first you can summarize what you need to do to bring yourself within the healthy physical activity guidelines described above.

Improving Your Cardio Training

☐ There's no need for me to change; I am within the recommended guidelines.

☐ I need to increase in the following ways: _____

_____

☐ I need to decrease in the following ways: _____

_____

Improving Your Strength Training

☐ There's no need for me to change; I am within the recommended guidelines.

☐ I need to increase in the following ways: _____

_____

☐ I need to decrease in the following ways: _____

_____

Improving Your Flexibility Training

☐ There's no need for me to change; I am within the recommended guidelines.

☐ I need to increase in the following ways: _____

_____

☐ I need to decrease in the following ways: _____

_____

FINDING THE RIGHT PHYSICAL ACTIVITIES FOR YOU

It is likely that you will only start, or continue with, physical activities that suit you and your lifestyle. Take a look at the following table to help you identify your preferences. Complete the first column, identifying your overall preferences right now. If your physical activity is in line with your life priorities, you are more likely to continue with the activity. Next, complete the second column to highlight the 3-5 priorities that are most important to you. For example, you may feel strongly that you want to spend more time with your family but not care about whether you are doing something familiar or trying something new. You would only check the row related to family.

Your Preferences (In each box, select one preference.)	Your Current Life Priorities (Select your top three to five priorities.)
☐ Be a leader	☐
☐ Learn from a teacher	☐
☐ Be competitive	☐
☐ Be noncompetitive	☐
☐ Have fun	☐
☐ Have a sense of accomplishment	☐
☐ Use my talents	☐
☐ Learn something new	☐
☐ Enjoy the outdoors	☐
☐ Enjoy an indoor setting	☐
☐ Be independent	☐
☐ Work with a team	☐
☐ Enjoy tranquility	☐
☐ Experience excitement	☐

☐ Feel challenged ☐ Feel safe and secure	☐ ☐
☐ Enjoy the familiar ☐ Try something new	☐ ☐
☐ Spend time on my own ☐ Spend time with others	☐ ☐
☐ Meet new people ☐ Spend time with family and friends	☐ ☐
☐ Have a structured approach ☐ Embrace variety and novelty	☐ ☐

Now that you have considered your life priorities or preferences, on the lines below write what seem to be your main priorities at this point in your life. List at least three.

_____

_____

_____

Matching Your Priorities to Specific Physical Activities

Consider the physical activities listed below and decide whether any of them would satisfy the priorities or preferences you identified above. The first column lists activities that require you to set time aside and are often (although not always) done independently. The second column lists activities that require you to belong to a team or play with a partner. The third column lists daily-living activities for people who want to build activity into their lifestyle and like to feel productive when they are active.

Make a check mark next to the items that appeal to you and match your priorities.

Planned Activities	Team/Pair Activities	Lifestyle Activities
☐ Aerobics	☐ Baseball	☐ Gardening
☐ Aquafit aerobics	☐ Curling	☐ Raking
☐ Gym machines	☐ Football	☐ Hand-mowing lawn
☐ Walking	☐ Golf	☐ Wood cutting
☐ Jogging/running	☐ Hockey	☐ Vacuuming
☐ Inline skating	☐ Racquetball	☐ Mopping
☐ Swimming	☐ Soccer	☐ Sweeping
☐ Hiking	☐ Tennis	☐ Scrubbing
☐ Cycling	☐ Volleyball	☐ Painting
☐ Ice skating	☐ Basketball	☐ Pushing stroller
☐ Dancing	☐ Squash	☐ Carrying groceries
☐ Kickboxing	☐ Fencing	☐ Dog walking
☐ Canoeing	☐ Ultimate Frisbee	☐ Hoeing
☐ Climbing	☐ Boxing	☐ Digging
☐ Horseback riding	☐ Dancing	☐ Stacking wood
☐ Skiing	☐ Canoeing	☐ Playing physical games with kids
☐ Weight training		
☐ Yoga		
☐ Martial arts		
☐ Tai chi		

Write down the physical activities you selected that you know you could take part in immediately:

_____

_____

Write down the physical activities you selected that you would need to research or prepare for before you could start:

_____

_____

Take one week to look into the activities that interest you and then move toward designing your plan, as described below.

GETTING SPECIFIC: DESIGNING YOUR PLAN

Whether you decide to set aside time for activity in your life or to work activity into your daily living, you are unlikely to make any changes unless you have a specific plan. At the top of each of the following tables is an example of a physical activity plan that could be built into a person's daily life. Fill in your plan below:

Cardio Activity

Time (Duration)	Activity
An example:	
Weekday:	
2 x 10 min.	*Walk to bus stop, briskly*
20 min.	*Walk at lunch*
20 min.	*Walk dog*
60 min.	**Total for Day**
Weekend:	
40 min.	*Basketball at local community center*
20 min.	*Walk dog*
60 min.	**Total for Day**
Your plan:	

Strength Training

Days per Week	Activity
An example: *2 days (Wed., Sat.)*	*Groceries (lift each bag twice)* *Vacuum* *Scrub tub*
Your plan:	

Flexibility

Days or Times per Week	Activity
For example: *When watching the news (every night)*	*Stretch in front of the television.*
Your plan:	

GETTING STARTED

Having a good plan is a big step toward getting started with physical activity. However, even with a good plan, you might never get started if you find ways to put it off. There's nothing like making a commitment to help you follow through. For some people, one effective form of commitment is to spend some money: buy yourself the equipment or clothing you will need for your chosen activity, pay to enroll in a class, or hire a personal trainer. Another way of making a commitment is to involve other people in your plans: find a friend who wants to start being active, choose an activity where people need you to be there (such as a sports team or doubles tennis), or join a group of people who are already active (such as a walking group). Finally, make a commitment of your time: set the date on which you will get started, and add the workout to your schedule and your calendar. Treat it like a mandatory work meeting or doctor's appointment. In other words, treat it with the importance it deserves.

Below, write the ways you will increase your commitment:

_____

_____

_____

_____

Before You Get Started: Some Final Words

Incorporating physical activity in your life is a crucial step toward improving your overall physical and psychological well-being. It's important, however, that you go about making this change safely. Talk with your doctor before you start becoming much more physically active. If you aren't feeling well, delay your activity plan until you feel well.

Janice had a busy personal and work life. She enjoyed meeting others, especially in her community. She was also eager for a few moments of tranquility in her life. She decided to join a local walking group led by a dynamic woman committed to the benefits of power walking. Janice felt she could quite easily keep up this activity while traveling, since most of the hotels she stayed in had treadmills that were available to guests. She also joined a weekly yoga class for strengthening, flexibility, and quiet.

Your Daily Plan Sheet

In chapter 5, you began to use a "Daily Plan" sheet to plan and track your eating. We have provided a similar sheet for you to use in planning and tracking your activity. Use both sheets on a daily basis until you feel that your eating and activity have settled into a healthy routine.

My Daily Plan and How I Am Doing

My activity plan for today (what kind of activity you plan to do, and where and when you will do it):	What I actually did today (describe the activity you did today):
Cardio What: Where: When: **Strength** What: Where: When: **Flexibility** What: Where: When:	**Cardio** What: Where: When: **Strength** What: Where: When: **Flexibility** What: Where: When:

My activity goal for today (for example, call the pool to find out schedule, park ten minutes away from work, stretch after walk at lunch):

What got in the way of my achieving my activity goal or following my plan (for example, circumstance, emotions, people, or other things):

CHAPTER CHECKLIST

You have completed this chapter when:

O   You have identified your physical and mental health reasons for being active.

O   You have calculated your working heart rate range.

O   You have evaluated your current level of fitness in the areas of cardio, strength, and flexibility.

O   You have determined the changes that you would have to make in order to cause your physical activity to fall within healthy guidelines.

O   You have considered your life and fitness priorities and chosen physical activities that match these priorities.

O   You have designed your own personal plan—describing the activities, duration of your activity, and what days of the week you will be active.

What do you do next and when?

O   Schedule an appointment with your family doctor to discuss your activity plan.

O   Start implementing the personalized activity plan that you have developed.

O   Move on to the chapters on overcoming obstacles when you have created both your eating plan (chapter 5) and your activity plan (this chapter).

O   Use the "Daily Plan" sheet to track your daily activity goals and record obstacles to meeting your activity goals. You will use this information when you work through the chapters on overcoming obstacles.

Deali[...]he Road

[handwritten annotation: CBT — Modifying what you think (cognition) And what you do (behavior) in response to the world around you.]

Having an eating and activity plan ready to go is a huge step toward living the healthy lifestyle you have chosen for yourself. The first weeks and months of putting your plan into place are full of challenges. This chapter will focus on some of the most common obstacles: the situational triggers. Chapters 8 and 9 will deal with the other triggers (emotional and interpersonal). The approach that we will use to these triggers is based on cognitive behavioral therapy (CBT). CBT is an evidence-based psychological treatment that aims to improve your emotional well-being and functioning by modifying what you *think* (cognition) and what you *do* (behavior) in response to the world around you.

IDENTIFYING YOUR PERSONAL TRIGGERS: SELF-MONITORING

The most powerful tool for discovering your personal triggers is self-monitoring. Self-monitoring involves tracking your own experiences so that you learn *exactly* what factors put you at risk. Once you know what your triggers are, you can use various strategies to reduce your risk of reacting to those triggers.

What Exactly Will You Be Monitoring?

In chapter 5, you wrote out your daily plan for eating and tracked what you actually ate. In this chapter, you are tracking the times when you *don't* follow your eating or activity plan for the day. For example, maybe you had a bad day and ate way more for dinner than you had planned. Maybe you skipped breakfast or canceled on your friend who was meeting you for your daily walk. These kinds of events are your cue to begin looking for the trigger that derailed your efforts. Once you know you are off track, you will follow the seven steps for self-monitoring, described below. We have illustrated each step using Jim's example.

Jim was talking with his doctor about weight-loss surgery and trying to follow the balanced deficit weight-loss plan in order to get used to more regular and balanced eating. He made his plan (three thousand calories, as calculated using the formulas in chapter 5) but ran into his first problem fairly quickly. Jim found that on the days his wife worked the night shift, he had to juggle more of the household tasks and his children's activities, leaving him little time to stick to his planned exercise or meals. On these days, he found himself falling back into old habits: forgoing physical activity and turning to fast food for dinner.

The Seven Steps of Self-Monitoring

Follow the steps below.

STEP 1: THE PROBLEM

When you review your day, you need to decide whether you followed your plan. You can only know this if you are clear on what you were planning for the day, so it's important to prepare your eating plan for the day and know what physical activity you intend to do. If you review your day and see many misses, you may want to work on only one or two things at a time. Start by focusing on something that's *almost* right. So, if all your meals and snacks didn't match what you planned, then you might start with the meal that came closest or that you think would be the easiest to fix. This meal is now your "problem," and you will think only of this as you fill in the rest of the steps.

Jim identified his problem as follows: "I didn't eat the dinner I had planned, and I didn't do the exercise I had scheduled for this afternoon."

STEP 2: THE SITUATION

The next thing that you need to track is your situation or circumstance at the time you had your "problem." Try to only discuss the circumstances and not your emotions or any interpersonal interactions that might have occurred (these will come next).

Jim described the situation by saying, "I was home alone with the kids because my wife is working nights this week. I was rushing around getting the girls to their soccer game and I had to pick up dog food because we were out, so I grabbed some fast food for dinner instead of cooking a healthy meal."

STEP 3: WHAT YOU FEEL

The next step is to identify the emotions you felt leading up to and at the time your "problem" occurred. You may have felt more than one emotion at the time. Chapter 8 will give you a complete list of possible emotions if you need help identifying what you feel. Note them all and rate each of them in intensity from 0 (not at all intense) to 100 (extremely intense). When you begin to work on emotional triggers, focus on the emotion that you rate the most intense.

Jim described his emotions by saying "I felt overwhelmed, stressed, and helpless," and he identified his feeling of being overwhelmed as the strongest emotion, with an intensity of 80 out of 100.

STEP 4: WHAT YOU THINK

The next step is to record what you were thinking. To get at the thoughts that will be the most useful, focus on the emotion you identified in step 3 as the most intense. Try to complete the following sentence: "I was feeling _____ [fill in the emotion that was most intense] because _____ [fill in the possible reason you felt that emotion].

Jim described his thoughts by saying, "I was feeling overwhelmed because I couldn't cope with all the demands on my own. I don't have enough time for all this. I'm never going to be able to do things for myself; my needs just don't take priority."

STEP 5: WHO ELSE IS INVOLVED?

In this step, you consider whether any personal interactions were related to the "problem" you identified. Consider whether any interactions occurred at the time of the problem, or if any past interactions might have put you at risk. Trust your mind to go to what's important; if something pops into your head, it might be of value in helping you to understand what has put you at risk.

Here are Jim's thoughts on his interpersonal triggers: "When I thought about what interactions might have contributed to missing my exercise, I found that the image of my wife popped into my head. This morning, when we talked about the plans for the day, she was exasperated when I mentioned my plans, and she said, 'Jim, you know the girls have soccer. There's nothing I can do about that now. I'm not home tonight. You have to take them.'"

STEP 6: WHAT YOU DO IN RESPONSE

The next step is to identify what you chose to do in response to the situation, your emotions, your thoughts, and the interactions you had with others.

Jim's response was as follows: "I guess I just accepted that I wouldn't be able to follow my plan. I put the kids' schedule first and dropped my plans for eating and physical activity."

STEP 7: WHAT YOU LEARNED

Ask yourself two questions:

1. *What put me most at risk?* This question helps you decide which type of trigger to focus on. Jim reviewed the different situational, emotional, and interpersonal information he had collected, and determined that it was mostly the situation that had put him at risk. "I guess when things get busy, I put my eating and physical activity at the bottom of the list."

2. *Is this situation likely to happen again?* This question helps you decide whether it's worth the effort to think ahead to times you will face this risk again. If you think the problem will happen again, it's worth coming up with a solution. Jim thought, "This is definitely going to happen again. I need to figure out how to deal with this situation."

Daily Eating, Activity, and Self-Monitoring Worksheet

In this chapter, we have expanded the daily planning sheet that you were given in chapter 5 to add the self-monitoring steps so you can identify the triggers that put you at risk for falling off your plan. Take a look at the Daily Eating, Activity, and Self-Monitoring Worksheet that follows. Photocopy the sheet for use each day or record the information in a notebook. Jim's worksheet is shown to illustrate what to record.

Daily Eating, Activity, and Self-Monitoring Worksheet

What I plan to eat today: (Fill in times, food choices, and amount.)	Food Servings*					Check if followed plan.	Check if ate less.	Check if ate more.
	G	F & V	D	M & A	F			
Wake-up time:								
Breakfast:								
Snack:								
Lunch:								
Snack:								
Dinner:								
Snack:								
Total Servings:								

My Activity Goal Today: **My Actual Activity:**

If I did not follow my plan today (or had the urge not to follow my plan), here's what happened:

1. Problem: _____

2. Situation: _____

3. What I felt: Emotion: _____ Intensity (0–100): _____

4. What I thought: _____

5. Who else was involved? _____

6. What I did in response: _____

7. What I learned: _____

* G = Grains, F & V = Fruits and veggies, D = Dairy, M & A = Meat and alternatives, F = Fats

Jim's Daily Eating, Activity, and Self-Monitoring Worksheet:

What I plan to eat today: (Fill in times, food choices, and amount.)	Food Servings*					Check if followed plan.	Check if ate less.	Check if ate more.
	G	F & V	D	M & A	F			
Wake-up time: *9:00 a.m.*						√		
Breakfast:								
2-serving bowl of cereal	2					√		
1 c. milk			1			√		
1 piece toast & 1 tsp. margarine	1				1	√		
2 scrambled eggs (w/1 tsp. margarine)				1	1	√		
Banana & ½ c. orange juice		2				√		
Snack: *None*								
Lunch: *Noon*								
Large kaiser bun	3					√		
3 slices ham				1		√		
1 sandwich-sized cheese slice			½			√		
1 tbs. low-fat mayo					1	√		
1 c. baby carrots & salad-dressing dip		2			1	√		
Apple		1				√		
Small yogurt			½					
Snack: *3:00 p.m.*								
1 serving crackers (according to label on box)	1						√	
1 ½ oz. cheddar cheese			1				*skipped*	
Apple		1						
Dinner: *6:30 p.m.*								
1 ½ c. rice	3							√
1 chicken breast (brushed w/olive oil)				1	1			*Ate*
1 small salad with light dressing		1			1			*fast food*
1 c. broccoli		2						*(lots)*
1 c. milk			1					
Snack: *9:30 p.m.*								
Trail mix (½ c. peanuts, ¼ c. raisins, 1 serving dry cereal)	1	1			3			
Total Servings:	11	10	4	3	9			

My Activity Goal Today: *Swim for 30 min.* **My Actual Activity:** *None*

If I did not follow my plan today (or had the urge not to follow my plan), here's what happened:

1. Problem: ___*Didn't eat planned dinner and didn't do the exercise I had planned*___

2. Situation: *Home alone, rushing the girls to their soccer game and had to pick up dog food*

3. What I felt: Emotion: ___*Overwhelmed*___ Intensity (0–100): ___*80*___

4. What I thought: *I felt overwhelmed because I can't cope with all these demands on my own.*

5. Who else was involved? ___*My wife was exasperated and said I had to take the girls to soccer.*___

6. What I did in response: ___*Focused on girls; dropped my eating and activity plans*___

7. What I learned: ___*I need a solution for when I'm busy. This will happen again.*___

When to Self-Monitor

Self-monitoring may seem straightforward and easy, but in practice it takes effort and commitment. To be successful, you must make time in your schedule each day to fill in your self-monitoring sheet. Ideally, you should record your eating throughout the day, right after you eat, especially because research suggests that our recall of food intake is not very reliable (Mulheim et al. 1998). At the least, make time each evening to record your eating as accurately as you can remember. Complete the bottom of the sheet whenever you check off the columns that indicate you ate less or more than you planned. You should also record when you have *urges* to get off track but manage to stay on track anyway. This will help you figure out what triggers make you vulnerable to slipping back into your old habits. Use the complete Daily Eating, Activity, and Self-Monitoring Worksheet (including the food you plan to eat) for your first month or two of following your new plan. When your eating feels more like a "habit"—in other words, you just know what's normal for you to eat for meals and snacks—then we suggest that you continue to use the bottom portion of the worksheet whenever you feel your eating or activity has gone off the rails.

PUTTING YOUR SELF-MONITORING TO WORK: FOCUSING ON YOUR TRIGGERS

So self-monitoring is going to help you identify the triggers that put you at risk for falling off your plan. So what? What do you do with this information? In this chapter and the two that follow, you will learn strategies for dealing with the situations, emotions, and interactions you identify as putting you and your plan at risk. The strategies you will learn will require you to actively pay attention to the triggers that make you vulnerable and then deal with them head-on. Active coping will ensure that you are successful with your goals.

In the final step of your self-monitoring process, you are asked to consider what you have learned. It is at this point that you decide which type of trigger caused you to depart from your plan: situational, emotional, or interpersonal. You may easily identify one type of trigger as the culprit. Alternatively, you may decide that more than one trigger needs to be addressed. For example, you may decide that you need to address situational factors (dealing with many food choices, for example) and emotional factors (your distress at seeing your ex-partner, for example) in planning ahead for your friend's potluck dinner. Once you identify the trigger you believe is responsible for pushing you off track, you need to decide whether you think this trigger is likely to be a problem again for you in the future. If you think you will run into this trigger again, then you will need to actively plan ahead for the next time. We will now focus on the most common trigger, the situational trigger.

Situational Triggers: Problem Solving and Planning Ahead

The solution for practical, everyday, situational problems relies entirely on common sense. You are simply going to apply yourself to the problem and see if you can come up with solutions that work; in other words, you will do some problem solving. You can do this when you find yourself in the middle of a problem, but it's more effective when you identify situations that put you at risk, and then plan ahead. We will take you through the problem-solving and planning-ahead process below and make suggestions that we hope will improve your chances of finding a successful solution. We will use Jim's example to illustrate the steps of problem solving.

Jim identified his busy schedule on the days his wife worked as the trigger for falling off his plan. Now that he had identified this situational trigger, Jim was motivated to find a better way of managing this situation. Before self-monitoring, he'd just thought he lacked willpower. Now that he had broken it down to a problem he could solve, it seemed more possible for him to stay on track with his eating and activity plan.

STEP 1: IDENTIFY THE PROBLEM

What's the problem that you need to address? How did you fall off your plan? This is the same as step 1 in your self-monitoring.

Jim identified two ways in which he fell off his plan:

1. *I didn't prepare and eat the dinner I planned.*

2. *I didn't do the physical activity I planned.*

STEP 2: CONSIDER ALTERNATIVE SOLUTIONS

What are possible ways that you can address your problem?

Under each problem, Jim wrote possible solutions.

1. *I didn't prepare and eat the dinner I planned.*

   Solutions:

   - *Choose a fast-food restaurant that offers healthy choices.*

   - *Pay for a meal service to deliver healthy meals.*

   - *Hire household help in order to free up time.*

   - *Make healthy meals ahead of time and put them in the freezer to pull out quickly when needed.*

   - *Plan out schedule in advance in order to build in time for meals.*

   - *Plan and prepare a meal I can take with me to eat on the go.*

2. *I didn't do the physical activity I had planned.*

   Solutions:

   - *Build physical activity into my day on these busy days; if I am at the soccer park, walk up and down the side of the field while the girls are at practice.*

   - *Arrange a carpool with other parents to free up time to exercise.*

   - *Get up forty-five minutes earlier in the morning to ride my exercise bike.*

When generating possible solutions, write down all the options that you can think of without limiting yourself. Then go through each possible solution individually and consider the following: What are the pros and cons? Is this solution realistic? Can this solution be implemented?

In reviewing each of his possible solutions, Jim realized that they really couldn't afford the options that required extra money, like hiring someone to help out or paying for a meal service. He didn't think he would have time to prepare a portable meal. He didn't think it was a good idea to rely on fast-food restaurants, as he was afraid he'd make a bad choice and was reluctant to spend money to eat out. In the end, he thought the best option would be to plan his meals ahead of time and freeze them so he could pull them out and heat them up quickly when things were hectic.

With respect to physical activity, Jim was worried that if he tried to build physical activity into his day, he wouldn't do very much at all—and he liked to chat with the other parents at the park. He also didn't like the carpool idea because then he would be obligated to reciprocate and that might add more pressure. He thought the idea of getting up early to ride his exercise bike seemed like the best option.

STEP 3: DEVELOP YOUR IMPLEMENTATION PLAN

Once you have considered the possible options and selected a solution, you need to develop a detailed implementation plan that addresses what you will do, how you will do it, when you will do it, and whether any other people will be involved.

In the week prior to his wife's shift change, Jim planned to make some meals that he could freeze (for example, a pot of soup and a casserole). Each of these items would be enough to feed the family for two dinners; once when he made them and a second time after freezing them. He planned to buy precut vegetables that could easily be taken out of the fridge for a quick snack or to accompany the meal. He also planned to make a special grocery trip for the week so that he could stock up on the ingredients that he needed as well as healthy convenience foods that they could eat with lunches or as snacks (for example, cold cuts, yogurts, trail mix, and fruit). Jim also planned to set his alarm forty-five minutes earlier so he would have time to get dressed and exercise. He discussed both plans with his wife. She was very supportive and offered to help with making the meals that they would freeze.

Step 3a: Developing a Fall-Back Plan. In reading through Jim's plan, you may be thinking "Wow, that sounds amazing, but can he really do it?" We would agree that Jim has chosen what might be considered the most "ideal" plan. Often, when problem solving, people feel compelled to plan what they think would be the ideal: healthy, home cooked, and inexpensive. If you think you can do this, we agree that you should give it a try. But in reality, any solution that requires a big change in routine or effort is difficult to implement or continue over time. Therefore, come up with a fall-back plan—something convenient that is close to what you were already doing. It is rarely your idea of perfection. Jim was reluctant to consider a less-than-ideal alternative, but he came up with the following plan:

Jim decided his fall-back plan would be one he had originally rejected. He decided that, should he and his wife falter in their commitment to prepare frozen meals, he would plan to choose healthier options at a fast-food restaurant. To minimize his risk of choosing old unhealthy favorites, he decided to choose a fast-food restaurant that mostly offered healthy choices (for example, a sub or pita restaurant). Although he felt it wasn't the ideal solution, he was confident he could rely on it; it was similar to his previous behavior and was certainly convenient.

For physical activity, Jim chose to walk the soccer field. It was convenient and didn't require a change of schedule. To increase his motivation, Jim decided to ask one of the other dads, one who always brought his dog, to join him in walking the field.

STEP 4: IMPLEMENT YOUR PLAN AND EVALUATE.

Once you have created your detailed implementation plan, it's time to put it into action and then step back and evaluate the results. Depending on how things go, consider whether you need to modify the plan for future use.

Jim found that he actually enjoyed cooking with his wife and feeling more in control of what he would be eating. It took quite a bit of effort and planning ahead, but the payoff was worth it. He struggled the first few days to get up at the earlier time to exercise, but he adjusted by going to bed a bit earlier the night before.

Jim did acknowledge that there might be times in their lives when it would be hard to keep up this level of preparation. He felt good about his efforts to follow his ideal plan, but he was reassured to know that he had a fall-back plan for more challenging times.

PROBLEM-SOLVING AND PLANNING-AHEAD WORKSHEET

Now it's time for you to plan ahead for and resolve the situational triggers you have identified through your self-monitoring. You may need to fill out the following worksheet many times over the first few weeks as you identify different situations that have interfered with your eating and activity plan. You can photocopy the blank worksheet and fill out the photocopies or record the answers in a notebook.

Problem-Solving and Planning-Ahead Worksheet

Problem: How did you fall off your plan? _____

Is this problem likely to occur again, and when? _____

Situational trigger contributing to the problem: _____

What are some possible solutions to this problem?

    Solution 1: _____

    Solution 2: _____

    Solution 3: _____

    Solution 4: _____

What are the pros and cons of each possible solution?

    Solution 1: _____

    Solution 2: _____

    Solution 3: _____

    Solution 4: _____

Which solution is the best fit for you? (Consider the pros and cons, and your ability to implement it.)

_____

Develop your implementation plan. Be as detailed as possible (what, how, when, where, and who):

_____

Once you implement your plan, think about how it went. Do you need to make any modifications?

_____

If things don't go according to plan, what's your fall-back plan?

_____

SITUATIONAL TRIGGERS THAT DESERVE SPECIAL ATTENTION

Some common situational triggers deserve special mention: foods that put you at risk for falling off your plan, where you eat your food, buffet eating or feasting, and your own biology (your body's need to eat enough food at regular intervals). When you are solving problems around these situational triggers, feel free to take advantage of some of the suggestions we provide.

Trigger Foods. Trigger foods are foods you just can't seem to eat in reasonable quantities. You arrive home to the smell of just-baked chocolate chip cookies. Your friend shows up to watch a movie and brings a bag of chips; he opens the bag and offers you some. These are examples of foods where one bite just seems to lead to the next, until all the food disappears.

Give some thought to the foods that seem to trigger your overeating, and make a list below:

_____

_____

_____

Your list may include both "treat" foods and foods that would be considered part of a healthy meal (for example, pasta, bread, or cheese).

In resolving how to handle trigger foods, consider the following suggestions:

- Limit your access to these foods. Keep them out of your home.

- When you *do* choose to eat these foods, try to plan things so that you only have access to the serving size you wish to eat. You may wish to stop at a convenience store to pick up one chocolate bar or one small bag of chips.

- If you have to buy treat foods for others in your home, try to choose foods that aren't your preference so you won't be as tempted.

- Only cook what you think will be eaten at that meal when preparing a trigger food.

- With "treat" foods, try to eat them when you have already eaten a meal or snack and aren't hungry. These foods are meant to bring pleasure into your life; they should not be relied on to alleviate hunger, if possible.

The Way You Eat: "Stimulus Control." We know that mindless eating is more likely to result in the consumption of larger quantities of food.

Give some thought to the circumstances in which you tend to eat your meals and describe each below:

Breakfast: _____

_____

Lunch: _____

_____

Dinner: _____

_____

Snacks: _____

_____

Now evaluate where you eat against the following recommendations:

■ When possible, eat your meals at the table.

■ Spend some time on the "presentation" of the meal: prepare a plate of food that looks attractive and balanced.

■ Try to savor your food. Enjoy the smell, the taste, and the texture of your food. Try not to rush when you eat.

■ When you are finished with your meal, leave the table and make yourself comfortable.

■ Don't snack or eat your meals in front of the television; this is the ultimate in mindless eating.

■ Don't snack or eat when driving in the car, working at the computer, or whenever you will only be partially concentrating on the pleasure of eating.

■ In general, try to eat in a circumstance and at a time when eating is the only focus so that you enjoy what you eat and don't mindlessly consume more than you intended.

Buffet Eating or Feasting Meals. Celebration feasts and buffet eating present the same challenges to your eating plan: there are many rich and palatable foods available in virtually unlimited quantities.

Give some thought to your lifestyle. How often do these types of meals occur? List the predictable ones below:

_____

_____

_____

The healthy living plan allows you to have two "exceptional" meals per week, which makes it possible for you to participate more fully in celebrations. If you are following the weight-loss plan, you would ideally continue to limit your food to the recommended portions, regardless of the circumstances. In either case, you don't want to lose control of your eating. Consider the following recommendations when you're faced with buffet or feasting meals:

■ Eat normally, following your usual plan before the feasting meal. "Saving up" for the feast only leaves you hungry and less in control.

- Check out all the food options before filling your plate.

- Try to follow your plan for general food group servings for the meal, but decide not to worry about preparation. In other words, your fat servings may be higher on these special days.

- Decide how you will participate in the celebration. If you are following the healthy living plan, you may decide to relax and not follow any guidelines for the event. If you follow your usual eating plan for the day, you won't be overly hungry when you start eating, and you are unlikely to gorge. It *would* be normal, however, to feel very full if you eat more than you usually do. If you are on the weight-loss plan, you may make a more modest concession; for example, decide to have a serving of any dessert you choose, regardless of whether it fits your plan.

- Try to enjoy the food. Take your time. Chat with people between servings.

- If possible, move to a food-free location once you are done eating.

- If you must stay at the table, order a tea or coffee so that you have something to sip on rather than continuing to nibble at the food.

Your Own Biology: Meeting Your Body's Needs. It may seem odd to put your own biology as a possible situational trigger. To be successful with your eating and activity plan, however, you must respect your body's rhythms and needs. If you ignore your body's needs, you risk losing control of your eating. Whether you are following the healthy living or the weight-loss plan, eat every three to four hours and meet your body's need for the quantity of food on your plan. If you ignore one or both of these recommendations, you are at risk of experiencing powerful hunger cues from your body, which put you at great risk for losing control over your eating. If you are following the weight-loss plan, your body is already on the edge of hunger, and you need to be particularly careful with both the timing and quantity of food you give yourself. We think this is particularly important to mention, because there are some people who restrict or eat very little food during the day, only to lose control in the late afternoon or evening. It is *essential* to the success of both plans that you distribute your food evenly throughout your waking hours.

Give some thought to times when you are at risk of either going for too long between snacks or meals or skipping them altogether. Describe these below:

_____

_____

_____

Consider the following recommendations as you solve problems around following your eating plan:

- Eat within an hour of waking, and eat no more than three to four hours apart after that.

- If you lose control of your eating, *always* check to see whether hunger could have been a contributing factor: did you go too long before eating, and did you eat all the food you had planned until that point? (Notice on Jim's worksheet earlier in this chapter that he skipped his afternoon snack, which may have increased his risk of overeating fast food later.)

- Are you meeting the goal of eating two thirds to three quarters of your food servings *before* dinner?

- Plan your day; set your watch to beep and remind you to eat at regular intervals.

- Don't cut back your food because you think you can lose weight even more quickly. If you did so, you would only increase the risk that you will fall off your plan completely.

IN CONCLUSION

In this chapter you learned about the situational triggers that can act as bumps in the road, taking you off track from your eating and activity plans. You learned how to self-monitor, which will help you to identify your personal triggers. You also learned how to manage situational triggers through planning ahead and problem solving. In the next two chapters, you will learn strategies for managing emotional and interpersonal triggers.

CHAPTER CHECKLIST

You have completed this chapter when:

O You have practiced self-monitoring and identified situational triggers that have thrown you off track while trying to reach your eating and activity goals.

O You have engaged in planning-ahead and problem-solving strategies in response to recurring situational triggers you identified from your self-monitoring.

What do you do next and when?

O Continue to practice self-monitoring using the Daily Eating, Activity, and Self-Monitoring Worksheet. Continue this strategy for the next few weeks or months, until you feel your eating is habitual. Following that, we recommend that you record your triggers whenever you slip or get off track while trying to reach your eating and activity goals.

O When you identify situational triggers, continue to use planning and problem solving to help you overcome the situational triggers you identify.

O You are now ready to go to chapter 8 and learn strategies for managing emotional triggers.

CHAPTER 8

Managing Emotional Triggers

This chapter explores the emotional triggers that may derail your eating and activity plan. Emotions serve an important purpose: they provide us with information, prepare us to respond to a situation, and influence our social behavior (Gross 1998). However, emotions are sometimes distressing, and you may have found that eating is one way of dealing with them. The purpose of this chapter is to help you identify, tolerate, and respond to emotions in ways that leave you feeling strong, in control, and effective.

UNDERSTANDING YOUR EMOTIONS FROM A COGNITIVE BEHAVIORAL THERAPY (CBT) PERSPECTIVE

Using a CBT approach, you can understand your emotional experience by breaking it down into five components:

The Situation

Identify the situation or circumstance that prompted your emotional response. It may be an external event (something that happened to you) or an internal event (a thought, memory, image, or bodily sensation). Below is an example of an external event.

Jennifer receives a voice mail message from a friend, who cancels their date for shopping without providing a reason.

Your Interpretation

This is the personal meaning you give to the situation, which you express through thoughts and beliefs. Consider the two possible interpretations below.

Example 1: *Jennifer thinks, "That's okay. Now I can work on my paper that's due next week."*

Example 2: *Jennifer thinks, "That sucks. Now I have nothing to do for the day."*

Your Body's Response

The experience of emotion is powerfully influenced by the sensations you feel in your body. These sensations can greatly intensify your emotional experience and even shape your interpretations of events. For example, "If I feel *this* aroused I must be *really* angry."

Example 1: *Jennifer's body feels light. She feels the release of muscle tension she wasn't aware of.*

Example 2: *Jennifer feels a hollowness in her chest, her throat tightening.*

Your Emotion

Emotions are our attempt to put a label on the combined experience of our interpretation of the situation and our bodily response.

Example 1: *Jennifer describes her emotions as "relief and happiness."*

Example 2: *Jennifer describes her emotions as "disappointment and loneliness."*

Your Behavioral Response

In response to your interpretation of the situation and your body's sensations, you experience an urge to act or behave in some way. Your behaviors can also intensify your emotional experience, reinforcing your interpretation of events.

Example 1: *Jennifer smiles and makes a plan for how she will now organize her day.*

Example 2: *Jennifer grabs a bag of chips, turns on the television, and tries to distract herself from her feelings of loneliness.*

BUT I'M NOT SURE WHAT EMOTION I'M FEELING!

As you can see, labeling an emotion requires a rather complex process of synthesizing information about your experience, your interpretation of the meaning of the experience, your bodily sensations, and your behavioral urges. Given the complex nature of this process, you may find it difficult to identify and label your emotions. You may have become accustomed to eating as a coping strategy, so you may no longer be aware of any preceding emotional trigger.

The first step in figuring out what emotion you are experiencing is to learn how to name your feeling. An emotion is often best captured in one word, as illustrated in the table below.

Joyful	Loved	Angry	Anxious	Sad	Ashamed
Excited	Adored	Mad	Scared	Depressed	Guilty
Amused	Liked	Irritated	Frightened	Down	Embarrassed
Happy	Cared for	Annoyed	Nervous	Hurt	Humiliated
Eager	Attractive	Frustrated	Worried	Dejected	Mortified
Interested	Desired	Enraged	Apprehensive	Lonely	Self-conscious
Curious		Furious	Terrified	Miserable	Regretful
Hopeful		Aggravated	Panicked	Despair	
Elated		Resentful	Stressed	Anguished	
Content			Overwhelmed	Rejected	
			Helpless		

Consider the information that you have gathered about your emotions from your self-monitoring, or think through other experiences you have had. List the emotions that may precede your getting off track from your eating and activity plan:

_____

_____

Monitoring the Five Components

For the next week, when you identify an emotional trigger on your Daily Eating, Activity, and Self-Monitoring Worksheet, practice observing your emotional experience and then break it down into the five components.

The Five Components of Emotional Experience				
Situation	Interpretation (What you think)	Body's Response (Physical sensations)	Emotion(s) (What you feel)	Behavioral Response (What you do)

COPING WITH YOUR EMOTIONS

CBT emphasizes the important role that your thoughts (or interpretations) and behaviors play in determining your emotional response to a particular situation. Two people can experience very different emotional responses to the same situation because of the different way they each interpret the situation. Consider the previous example of Jennifer and how she responded to her friend's canceling their shopping plans. When she interpreted the situation as positive because it left her some unexpected free time to work on her studies, she felt happy and experienced some stress relief. In contrast, when she interpreted the situation as a social rejection leaving her with nothing to do, she felt disappointed and lonely. The important message here is that, although you may think that you are having an emotional response to a situation, in fact your emotional response is greatly determined by your thoughts or interpretation of the situation. As you will see, examining your thoughts is an important key to changing your emotional response.

Your behaviors are also very important, because they can serve to increase or decrease the intensity of your emotions as well as modify how you think about the situation. When Jennifer interpreted the situation as positive, she responded by making an action plan for how she would use this time. This action probably led her to feel more in control. In contrast, when she interpreted the situation as a social rejection, she felt down and responded by crashing on the couch in front of the television with her comfort food. This behavioral response likely led her to feel worse and may have triggered further negative thoughts like "Great, now I have messed up my eating plan too. I'm a loser." You can see how behaviors can affect both your thoughts and your mood.

Keeping Your Emotions on an Even Keel: Are Your Thoughts Realistic?

Sometimes it's reasonable to feel anxious, down, angry, or embarrassed. In these cases, you are usually faced with a real problem that needs your problem-solving skills (as you learned in chapter 7). Sometimes, however, you can suffer with these emotions when suffering isn't warranted. The strategies we will teach you are intended to help you examine the thoughts that drive your emotional experience, with the goal of keeping you on a more even keel so you can more effectively use those problem-solving skills. We will target your thoughts with two goals in mind: enhancing your ability to see situations from a range of perspectives, and increasing your ability to develop balanced and realistic thoughts about a situation.

As you experience a negative emotion, you will practice stepping back and taking a look at what's going on by following the steps below:

STEP 1

Identify the emotion you have difficulty with. Earlier in this chapter, you were asked to identify the emotions from your self-monitoring that triggered you to overeat or fall off your plan. Start here by identifying one emotion you feel you particularly struggle with:

STEP 2

Pick a specific situation where this emotion triggered you to overeat or not stick to your eating or activity plan. Go through your self-monitoring and describe one such situation:

_____

STEP 3

Rate the intensity of the emotion you felt at the time (0 means not intense at all; 100 means extremely intense): I would rate my emotion at _____ out of 100.

STEP 4

Write out the thoughts that were associated with the emotion. Try to imagine feeling the emotion again. Fill in the blanks: *I felt... because...*:

_____

_____

_____

_____

You may have more than one thought. Try to make sure that all your thoughts relate to the situation you described in step 2. If you make a generalization about yourself ("I'm a loser"), make sure you relate it to the situation ("I'm a loser because I forgot to pack my lunch"). If your thought is in question form ("What if I fail?"), rewrite it as a statement ("I'm going to fail"). Try to be as specific as possible in describing your thoughts.

Step 5: Pick the thought that seems most powerfully related to the emotion. Write it below and rate how strongly you believe this thought:

_____

I rate my belief in this thought at _____ out of 100.

STEP 6

Write out the evidence that supports your thought. Stay with your emotion and your thought, and write down all the things you can think of that support your thought. Write the evidence below:

_____

_____

_____

_____

STEP 7

Now, write out all the evidence against your thought. In this step, we want you to switch gears. Try to think of any points that could be used to argue against your thought (the one you wrote in step 5). Consider what you would tell a friend who had that thought. Look at your evidence in step 6 and see if you could argue against that evidence. Write your arguments against the thought below:

_____

_____

_____

STEP 8

Review the evidence for and against, and come up with a "balanced" thought. Here, try to consider both sides and summarize the evidence for and against. See if you can write a balanced thought below:

_____

_____

Rate how much you believe this thought (0 means you don't believe it at all; 100 means you believe it completely): I believe it _____ out of 100.

STEP 9

Reevaluate your thought in step 5 and your emotion in step 3.

How much do you believe your thought now? _____ out of 100.

How strong is your emotion now? _____ out of 100.

STEP 10

What action do you need to take? If you found your thought to be realistic and your emotion is unchanged, then you likely have a realistic problem that needs to be solved. If you found that your thought and emotion changed over the course of this exercise, you may want to consider what you want to do from here. Write out your action plan below:

_____

_____

_____

YOUR THOUGHT RECORD

We have given you the following Thought Record worksheet so that you can work through your thoughts whenever you find that emotions seem to be triggering you to overeat or give up on your activity goals. Photocopy this blank form and use it as you need it. Remember, the Thought Record won't necessarily magically transform your emotions; what they will do is help you be certain that your emotions are based on a realistic interpretation of events. We have also given you Jennifer's thought record as an example.

Jennifer and her boyfriend had been invited to a party. On the day of the party, Jennifer was feeling tired and down, so she told her boyfriend she didn't feel up to going. He became quite angry and stormed out to go on his own. Normally, this kind of situation would have led her to give up on her plan and eat for comfort. But when she worked through the Thought Record, her mood changed and she felt less anxious and needing to eat.

For the next week, complete the Thought Record each time an emotional trigger gets in the way of your ability to meet your eating and activity goals.

Thought Record

Situation: Describe the situation leading up to the emotional trigger.

_____

_____

Emotion: Describe the emotion and rate its intensity. If you have more than one emotion, pick the one you want to work on first. Often this is the one with the highest rating.

_____ Rating: _____out of 100

_____ Rating: _____out of 100

_____ Rating: _____out of 100

Thought: Describe the thoughts related to the emotion you have chosen to work on. Make sure the thought is connected to the emotion you are focusing on and not one of the others you identified.

_____

_____

_____

Choose the thought above that you think is most powerfully related to your emotion and rate your belief in the thought here:

_____ out of 100.

Evidence For: List the evidence supporting your thought.

_____

_____

_____

Evidence Against: List the evidence against your thought.

_____

_____

_____

Balanced Thought: Summarize the evidence for and against your thought.

_____

Action Plan: What do you need to do?

_____

Jennifer's Thought Record

Situation: Describe the situation leading up to the emotional trigger:

Steve and I had a fight because I don't want to go out with him to the party.

Emotion: Describe the emotion and rate its intensity. If you have more than one emotion, pick the one you want to work on first. Often this is the one with the highest rating.

Anxious Rating: *80* out of 100 * *(I pick this one.)*

Depressed Rating: *75* out of 100

Mad Rating: *50* out of 100

Thought: Describe the thoughts related to the emotion you have chosen to work on. Make sure the thought is connected to the emotion you are focusing on and not one of the others you identified.

He's going to leave me because I'm so much trouble.

He won't love me anymore. * (This is the most powerful thought.)

He's never going to understand.

Choose the thought above that you think is most powerfully related to your emotion and rate your belief in the thought here:

80 out of 100.

Evidence For: List the evidence supporting your thought.

We fight all the time about this. He thinks it's ridiculous that I'm so worried about my appearance. There are lots of girls he could choose from who don't have this problem. He was really mad when he left.

Evidence Against: List the evidence against your thought.

We don't fight about anything else; we normally get along really well. He knows I'm working to change things, and he's usually supportive. He thinks my worries are ridiculous; he says he loves the way I look. When we're together he tells me he loves me and we talk about our future together.

Balanced Thought: Summarize the evidence for and against your thought.

My not wanting to go out is a real problem for us, but otherwise we are good and I know he loves me.

Action Plan: What do you need to do?

I need to make it a priority to work on this, and I need to talk to Steve so he knows I'm trying.

COUNTERING NEGATIVE THOUGHTS ABOUT EMOTIONS

In the previous section, we focused on your thoughts in response to how you felt. Now, we want to focus on your thoughts about feelings themselves. If you grew up in a household where emotions weren't acknowledged or were considered a weakness of character, then you may hold negative beliefs about experiencing emotions. Research has shown that negative evaluation of your emotional expression through self-criticism or negative judgments (such as telling yourself that you are stupid for feeling a particular way) can have a detrimental effect on your well-being (Low, Stanton, and Bower 2008). In fact, when you judge a feeling to be unacceptable and engage in behaviors to control or avoid it, you actually increase your emotional distress (Hayes, Strosahl, and Wilson 1999). In order to deal with your emotions effectively, take a stance of openness and acceptance toward your feelings and observe them in a non-judgmental fashion; this approach will help you to respond in a healthy and effective way (Campbell-Sills et al. 2006).

To become a good observer of your emotional experience, you will need to examine and challenge the negative, self-critical, or judgmental thoughts you have about emotional experiences.

Record these thoughts in the Negative Thought column below. Then practice countering each thought. Consider what you would say to a friend or a child who had that thought. What would a friend say to you if you told them you had that thought?

Negative Thought	Countering Thought
Showing emotion means I'm weak.	*My emotions are important signals. They are not a sign of weakness, as my father always led me to believe. In fact, it takes a lot of personal strength to face my emotions head-on.*
If I let myself experience a negative emotion, it may never turn off and I'll become paralyzed.	*Although I'm afraid of becoming completely paralyzed by my emotions, I'm willing to try and see what happens. That's the only way I can practice managing how I feel. Emotions usually pass on their own.*

If you have trouble generating countering thoughts, consider some of these possibilities:

■ Emotions are like the ocean. They are never static. Although they may come on intensely during a strong tide, they will also recede. I just need to wait the emotion out.

■ I can tolerate a strong emotion. It won't overwhelm me, even though I may feel as if it will.

■ My emotion is a message to me. I need to use my strong emotion as an opportunity to learn about myself and deal more effectively with what's going on in my life.

■ Although eating may temporarily make me feel better, it won't address the real issue, and just makes things worse for me in the long run.

Changing Your Behaviors

Sometimes your emotions are so intense that you can't imagine sitting down to complete the Thought Record. Maybe you need to be comforted or distracted in order to deal with intense emotions. If you usually turn to food to cope in these situations, then you need some alternative options. Although managing your emotions with food may work effectively for you by providing immediate relief or enjoyment, this strategy will be a major barrier against your efforts to make permanent changes in your life. This section provides you with a variety of strategies aimed at changing up your behavioral responses to emotional challenges. These strategies may not be as fast acting as food, but they will help you to stay on track with your eating and activity goals. The strategies are organized according to the different functions that food may have played in helping you to manage your emotions. Read the sections that are personally relevant to you. Remember, you don't know if a strategy will work if you haven't tried it!

As you struggle to cope with intense emotions, it's helpful to remember that emotions are like waves: they rise, they peak, and they inevitably fall in intensity. We are probably best able to think clearly when the intensity of an emotion is low, either as the emotion is beginning to rise or after it has peaked and begun to fall in intensity. You may need some help getting through the peak of an emotion so that you can actually complete the Thought Record or solve the problem. Even if you have found the Thought Record to be helpful, it may take you a while to settle down emotionally, and this also requires some strategies. Just remember two things as you go through a difficult emotional experience:

■ The emotion will eventually pass. It cannot remain at the highest intensity forever.

■ As unpleasant as emotions can be, they will not harm you.

IF YOU EAT TO CALM YOURSELF WHEN YOU ARE AGITATED

Different emotions act as triggers for different people. For some people, it's when they are angry that they feel a strong urge to eat. For others, it happens when they are anxious or stressed. When you feel agitated, eating can be very calming. The trouble is that, though it works in the short run, it often leaves you feeling distressed in the long term.

For Jennifer, anxiety often triggered her to eat. After her fight with her boyfriend, she worked through her thoughts using the Thought Record. Although she then felt much more optimistic about the relationship, her anxiety was not completely gone—and it likely wouldn't be until she sorted things out with Steve. She was still vulnerable to the urge to eat to calm herself down and needed a strategy for coping.

Strategies to Ease Agitation

Think of a time when you ate because it helped to calm intense emotions. Describe below:

_____

Work on solutions (using the Problem-Solving and Planning-Ahead Worksheet from chapter 7) for reducing your risk during these vulnerable times. Below, write out the solutions you plan to try:

_____

_____

How can you calm yourself when you are agitated so that you can complete the Thought Record or solve your problems? Choose some strategies you think might work:

_____

_____

If you are having difficulty, you may want to try physical activity (go for a walk, a bike ride, or a swim), vigorous cleaning (scrub your floor or vacuum your house), or distracting yourself with phsysical sensations (take a cold or hot shower, or listen to loud music).

Jennifer worked on solving her problems and decided to go for a vigorous walk to deal with the anxiety she felt, until she had a chance to talk with Steve. She chose to study for her exams in the library, away from food.

IF YOU EAT TO COMFORT YOURSELF

When you eat for comfort, you may not "lose control" of your eating as much as choose eating as a strategy for coping with the emotions you are experiencing. People who engage in this type of emotional eating emphasize the comfort they get from food, and they worry that nothing else will work as well as food does in providing them with emotional relief. There are disadvantages to this strategy for coping with emotions. First, people who use this strategy continue to worry about their excessive eating and the impact it's having on their health. Second, you lose out on the valuable information that your emotions may be providing to you; if you cannot reflect on what you feel and why, you are doomed to find yourself in the same pattern over and over again.

Strategies for Gaining Comfort

Think of a time when you ate to comfort yourself. Describe below:

_____

When you delayed eating, what emotion(s) did you notice?

_____

Were you able to determine what was going on in your life that contributed to these emotions? Write the underlying problems below:

_____

_____

Use the Planning-Ahead and Problem-Solving Worksheet from chapter 7 and write the solutions you intend to try below:

_____

_____

While you work at addressing the underlying issue, you may need to find other ways of soothing yourself. Focus on each of your different senses (except taste) and see if you can come up with three things you would find soothing.

Things to look at that you find soothing:

1.

2.

3.

Things to listen to that you find soothing:

1.

2.

3.

Things to smell that you find soothing:

1.

2.

3.

Things to touch that you find soothing:

1.

2.

3.

Once Karen experimented with "observing" her emotional experience in a nonjudgmental way, she realized that she often became depressed when she felt lonely and isolated. In fact, when she took a step back and examined her life, she realized that since her divorce she had really withdrawn from many relationships, particularly because her friends were mostly people she had met with her husband. Karen became determined to establish some new social connections. She joined a scrapbooking club that her neighbor belonged to, and found that she enjoyed meeting new people.

IF YOU EAT TO DISTRACT YOURSELF

There are times when you may simply want a distraction from your emotional state. Perhaps the most common reason for eating to distract yourself is to cope with boredom. People who eat to distract themselves don't always feel that eating is a choice; they say it's very hard to resist eating when they are bored. There's no problem with wanting to distract yourself from boredom. The goal is to find distracting activities that contribute to your well-being. We want you to find a solution that works well both in the short term *and* in the long term.

Jim used food as a way of distracting himself from being bored on his night shift at work as well as a means to stay awake when he felt tired. It was an easy way to make it through the shift, but the foods he snacked on were usually treat foods like potato chips and chocolate bars.

Strategies to Manage Boredom

If you often eat in response to boredom, it's likely that you need to make some changes in your life in order to make your free time more interesting and engaging.

What activities or plans can you build into your life that will give you some direction or interest? Think of three things that you can do, and list them below:

1. _____

2. _____

3. _____

If you are stuck for ideas, consider some of the options below.

☐ Enroll in an interesting class (stained glass, woodworking, astronomy).

☐ Develop a new hobby (scrapbooking, bird-watching, cycling, photography).

☐ Join a club (walking club, tennis club, naturalist club, book club, bowling club).

☐ Volunteer at a local nonprofit or homeless shelter.

☐ Make some new friendships (through one of the activities above, or ask someone you know out for coffee or a movie).

☐ Consider a career or job change.

☐ Learn a new skill (a sport or hobby).

☐ Get a membership to your local art gallery or museum.

☐ Read a book on a topic you are unfamiliar with.

☐ Form your own club. Invite a few friends or neighbors to join you in a monthly activity (such as wine tasting, book reading, walking, or movie watching).

Jim ate to relieve boredom at work. He did some thinking about ways he could cope with his work environment that didn't involve food. He decided to talk with his boss about courses he might take that would improve his advancement opportunities. His boss suggested a leadership-skills course. Jim really enjoyed the material and felt much more energized about his job. In addition, not only did his snacking diminish, but he was much happier with his quality of life.

IF YOU EAT TO REWARD YOURSELF

Many people use food as a way to reward themselves. After all, what celebration doesn't involve food? This becomes a problem when you are using food as a way to reward yourself on a regular basis. If you wish to successfully follow your eating plan, you'll need to find other ways of rewarding yourself than food.

Carlos realized he was using food as a reward for himself for making it through another stressful day at his job as a school vice principal. Although he had always enjoyed his cooking hobby, he hadn't realized how much he was rewarding himself with decadent, rich foods as a way to feel better.

Strategies for Rewarding Yourself

It's understandable that food may have become a powerful reward for you: food tastes good, makes you feel good, and is easily accessible. However, if you have identified that you are using food as a reward on a regular basis, then it's important that you find alternative ways to reward yourself. These alternatives may not be as powerful or as quick acting but, in the long run, will help you to stay on course with your lifestyle goals.

Consider some other potential rewards for yourself and record three options below:

1. _____

2. _____

3. _____

If you are stuck for ideas, consider any rewards that you have enjoyed in the past that weren't related to food. Or, ask some friends what they use to reward themselves. If you are still stuck for ideas, consider some of the possibilities below:

☐ Buy yourself a new outfit.

☐ Make a date with a friend to see a new movie or show.

☐ Make a spa appointment.

☐ Take some time to read a good book.

☐ Plan a vacation.

You may also wish to examine the overall quality of your life. For example, if your work life is mostly stressful and offers you little reward, this might explain why you are looking for rewards through food. You may need to make some more significant changes to your life to make it more intrinsically rewarding.

If you are rewarding yourself with food, what are the reasons that your daily activities aren't rewarding in themselves? Describe below:

_____

_____

Use the Planning-Ahead and Problem-Solving Worksheet from chapter 7 to see if you can come up with some ideas for making your daily life more rewarding. Write the solutions you intend to try below:

_____

_____

Carlos didn't plan on giving up his hobby, but he did plan on trying new ways to cook food that fit with his lifestyle and eating goals. Upon reflection, he realized that he needed to find ways to make his work life more rewarding. He planned to talk to the principal at his school about spending less time dealing with student discipline and complaining parents, and more time working on teachers' professional development programs. If that didn't work, Carlos would seriously consider returning to classroom teaching, where he could enjoy working with the kids, away from the administrative hassles. In the meantime, Carlos also thought he might look into taking a weekend cooking course as a reward for dealing with his difficult job during the week.

SUMMING THINGS UP

In this chapter, you learned to understand your emotional experience from a CBT perspective. You have developed your skills at identifying and managing your emotional triggers using strategies to target both your thoughts and your behavioral responses. Remember, emotions serve an important function in keeping you in tune with yourself and what's around you. Although it's difficult, addressing your emotions head-on will be beneficial to your psychological well-being in the long run.

CHAPTER CHECKLIST

You have successfully completed this chapter when:

○ You understand that your emotions serve an important purpose, and you can step back and observe what's happening when you experience strong emotions.

○ You have practiced breaking your emotional experiences down into the five components.

○ You have practiced using the Thought Record in response to emotional challenges for at least one week, and you have challenged your negative beliefs about experiencing emotions.

○ You have practiced changing up your behavioral responses to problematic emotions that have triggered you to engage in emotional eating in the past.

What do you do next, and when?

○ Continue to practice self-monitoring using the Daily Eating, Activity, and Self-Monitoring Worksheet. Continue this strategy for at least the next six months, and even beyond that whenever you get off track from your eating and activity goals.

○ Whenever you identify situational triggers, continue to use the planning and problem-solving strategies you learned in chapter 7.

○ Whenever you identify emotional triggers, use the Thought Record and behavioral strategies for dealing with emotional eating.

○ You are now ready to move on to chapter 9, which will deal with interpersonal triggers.

CHAPTER 9

Managing Interpersonal Triggers

As you try to put your eating and activity plans into place, it may become painfully clear that you are surrounded by people who have their own eating and activity habits and opinions. Sometimes, the people you hope will support you end up standing in your way. If you live with other people, their eating habits can threaten to derail your efforts to change your lifestyle. Family and friends may criticize your efforts or tell you that what you are doing isn't working. Acquaintances and strangers can feel entitled to make comments or give suggestions. Even health care professionals can challenge your efforts to live in a healthy way. To stay on track with your plan, you may need to learn how to stand up for yourself. This chapter will help you do this while preserving both your relationships and your self-respect.

IDENTIFYING THE PROBLEM: WHO IS IN THE WAY?

We hope that it's immediately obvious to you who stands in your way. The things that they say and do make it difficult for you to follow your plan. In the self-monitoring you completed in chapter 7, did you notice that interactions with certain people in your life seem to derail you?

List these people below:

_____

_____

_____

_____

THREE TYPES OF INTERPERSONAL OBSTACLES

Three types of interpersonal problems might get in the way of you staying on your plan.

Interference and Sabotage

Interference happens when people close to you test your ability to follow your lifestyle plan; they may do this unintentionally. For example, your roommates may enjoy snacking on potato chips in the evening while watching television, and you may find it difficult to resist joining in. Sabotage is what happens when someone close to you knows of your efforts and deliberately disregards them. Sometimes they do this with good intentions. For example, your partner brings you a gift of chocolates, even though you have asked that tempting foods be kept out of the home. Sabotage may also occur when a person close to you puts his priorities ahead of yours. For example, your partner picks up fast food most nights because it's convenient even though you are trying to make healthier food choices.

The list below is based on factors that weight-control experts believe contribute to people's lack of success in following a healthy lifestyle plan. Depending on whether you have chosen to follow a weight-loss or healthy-living plan, you may find that some items are more relevant to you than others. Consider the list below and make a check mark next to the ways that you feel your partner, roommate, coworker, or other companion interferes with your lifestyle plan.

- ☐ Objects to eating meals at the table with you and prefers to eat in front of the television

- ☐ Won't participate in preparation of home-cooked meals and prefers to eat out

- ☐ Regularly snacks on "treat foods" in front of you and offers you some

- ☐ Regularly tells you that you shouldn't eat treat foods, even after you explain that they are part of your plan

- ☐ Skips meals and doesn't support your efforts to eat at regular times

- ☐ Prepares or serves very large portions, regardless of what you ask for

- ☐ Gives you a smaller portion than you request, for "your own good," challenging your control of your own food intake

- ☐ Encourages seconds regardless of your preferences

- ☐ Denies you seconds even when you know you are following your plan

- ☐ Prepares rich foods frequently, regardless of your preferences

- ☐ Gives you rich or high-calorie food as a "gift" or as a sign of affection

- ☐ Refuses to give you, and tells others not to give you, rich or high-calorie foods—despite your explanation that you can include these in your plan in moderation

☐ Schedules other events over the time you usually work out

☐ Complains about the time you "waste" working out

☐ Backs out of plans to be physically active together

☐ Expresses frustration with your efforts to build activity into your daily life

☐ Asks you to make exceptions to your efforts to build activity into your daily life for their convenience (for example, park closer to your destination, take the elevator, and so on)

You may have thought of other ways that people are interfering with your plan as you worked your way through the list above. Using the list above and your own experiences, identify who does what in interfering with your plan on the lines below. We have provided an example on the first line.

*My husband*_____ does this: *always brings snack foods home to eat at night.*_____

_____ does this: _____

_____ does this: _____

_____ does this: _____

Janice had completed her self-monitoring sheets for a few weeks and noticed one interpersonal situation that regularly pushed her off her plan. As you will remember, Janice had decided to try the weight-loss plan because of her family's history of heart disease. Before she began the plan, she and her husband ate healthy meals, but they snacked together on chips in the evening. Although Janice was trying to change her eating habits, her husband looked forward to their evenings of television and snacking. Janice didn't want to impose her lifestyle changes on her husband, so she initially tried to resist snacking. Despite her intentions, Janice often found herself giving in to temptation and eating the chips with her husband. She was beginning to think she needed to talk to her husband.

Attacking Your Self-Esteem

People close to you and complete strangers alike can attack your self-esteem through the things they say and do. People who are overweight or obese are likely to have high self-esteem when they take a certain view of weight and body image. In a review of the research literature, C. Johnson (2002) highlighted five factors that appear to protect the self-esteem of a larger person. For each of these factors, we describe ways that people in your life might threaten your self-esteem. Check those that apply to you.

1. People who are larger and who have good self-esteem do not view other overweight people with dislike, disapproval, or disgust.

   People in your life threaten your nonjudgmental view of overweight people by:

   ☐ Speaking about overweight people with disgust or disapproval

□ Making critical comments about other people based on their weight

□ Commenting on a person's weight as an important factor in their opinion of the other person

2. People who are larger and who have good self-esteem do not see everything, including their weight, as being under their personal control or as something deserved.

   People in your life threaten your ability to avoid self-blame by:

□ Telling you that you are clearly doing something wrong or you wouldn't be overweight

□ Telling you that you really should do something about your weight, implying it's completely under your personal control

□ Giving you advice about what you should do to "fix" your weight

3. People who are larger and who have good self-esteem do not base their opinions of themselves on what other people think.

   People in your life threaten your own positive view of yourself by:

□ Telling you that you *should* care about what others think

□ Telling you what others must think about you

□ Telling you the negative things they have heard others say about larger people

4. People who are larger and who have good self-esteem are able to see negative weight-related comments and behaviors as a form of prejudice, rather than believe that the problem lies with themselves.

   People in your life threaten your ability to recognize prejudice and not take it personally by:

□ Talking as if it is justified that larger people be treated badly

□ Encouraging you to lose weight or to hide rather than fight back when people treat you badly

□ Not standing up for you or others when people make critical remarks based on weight

5. People who are larger and who have good self-esteem are able to challenge society's view of attractive body types.

   People in your life threaten your ability to challenge society's view of body types by:

□ Encouraging you to wait until you lose weight before you buy nice clothes

□ Encouraging you to read fashion magazines or watch makeover or similar shows on television

□ Talking about their dislike of their own body or weight

While completing the above checklist, you may have thought of other ways in which people around you negatively affect your self-esteem. Write them below; we have provided an example on the first line:

_My mother_____ does this: _comments on a person's weight when talking about her._____

_____ does this: _____

_____ does this: _____

_____ does this: _____

Jennifer had noticed that her mother was a significant trigger for her. Jennifer's mother had her own concerns about appearances and weight, and had often suggested to Jennifer that they diet together. Jennifer had decided to follow the healthy-living plan but found herself tempted to either cut back her food intake or binge-eat after spending time with her mother. After completing her self-monitoring, she realized that even when her mother wasn't talking about Jennifer's weight, she was commenting on the weight and appearance of others. Jennifer recognized that this fueled her own insecurities about her weight and shape. She needed to address the issue with her mother.

Other Problems

It is possible that you are dealing with interpersonal problems that have nothing to do with your lifestyle plan or weight-related self-esteem. In some cases, it may be helpful to speak to the person to resolve your difficulties. In other cases, the problem may be more complex and you may require more support than we can provide in this book. If you believe that the relationship itself is in trouble or that asserting your needs poses a risk for you, then we advise you to seek advice from your physician or a counselor.

If you think that the relationship is generally a good one, but the person is doing something that bothers you, then the tools we provide below may be of use to you. In this case, write down the person's name and the nature of the problem:

_My roommate_____ does this: _stays up late, playing her music and keeping me awake. I'm so tired_

and frustrated that I just can't think about anything else.

_____ does this: _____

_____

_____ does this: _____

_____

_____ does this: _____

_____

GETTING YOUR NEEDS MET

There are a number of ways you might respond to feeling that your needs are being ignored or stepped on. If you've let your resentment build up long enough, you might explode in anger, saying or doing things you regret. Or, you might show your resentment in a less direct way, communicating your anger through silence or lack of responsiveness. You might swallow your needs, perhaps literally in food. Ideally, however, you find a way to effectively communicate your needs in a manner that's respectful toward the other person and leaves you feeling good about yourself. This is what we call being "assertive." Assertiveness is not aggressive—demanding, overbearing, or disrespectful—toward the other person. Nor is it passive—treating yourself and your needs as being unimportant. There are three basic goals of assertiveness:

- To communicate your needs clearly, so that you are understood

- To communicate your needs respectfully, without any "sting," so that the relationship is protected

- To communicate your needs with self-control and dignity, so that you leave the interaction with self-respect

How Do You Assert Your Needs?

We are going to spend quite a bit of time helping you prepare a "script" for asserting yourself with another person. However, before people try this more direct method of communicating their wishes, they may try some indirect means of communicating their wishes or needs. Indirect communication can be thought of as "hinting" at your needs. The advantage of hinting is that you don't communicate any displeasure on your part, and the other person is therefore unlikely to become defensive. The disadvantage is that the other person might much more easily disregard your hint. Let's start by looking more closely at hinting.

INDIRECT COMMUNICATION: HINTING

There are three approaches to hinting, and you may wish to combine them all in your attempt to communicate indirectly.

Janice was keen to try a less direct approach to changing her husband's behavior. In general, she felt he was sensitive to being told what to do, so she wanted to try to shape his behavior without being seen as telling him what to do. If this didn't work, she would try a more direct approach.

Read through the three approaches to hinting below, using Janice as an example. You will recall that Janice's husband was bringing snack foods home at night, and she had a hard time not joining him in eating the snacks.

1. Tell a positive story about another person and suggest that this might work well for you.
   Janice tells her husband about a friend who has been trying to make healthier choices at night and who has switched to eating cut vegetables with dip instead of the usual chips.

2. Set up the situation so that the behavior you desire is more likely to occur.
   Janice stops off at the local grocery store and buys some cut veggies and dip. That night, she puts the veggies and dip out and offers some to her husband.

3. Compliment the behavior you desire.
   Janice thanks her husband for joining her in eating the veggies and dip she prepared, and tells him how much this has helped her stick to her eating plan that day.

Thinking of the problem situations you have identified for yourself, write any ideas for indirectly communicating your wishes or needs:

_____

_____

_____

Remember that hinting sometimes doesn't result in the changes you hoped for. Try not to be angry with the other person. You may simply need to be more direct. The other person may not be picking up on what you want or need. Take a look at the section below on direct communication.

DIRECT COMMUNICATION: CREATING AN ASSERTIVENESS SCRIPT

Follow the steps below to create an assertiveness script.

Step 1: Start by trying to understand the other person's perspective. *Why* might that person behave that way? This can be a challenging step if you feel very angry with the other person. However, it's an essential step toward keeping the other person from reacting defensively; it shows that you have tried to understand that person's point of view. Maybe, in trying to understand the other person's point of view, you will find yourself less angry and therefore better able to communicate respectfully and effectively.

Following are two examples of people trying to understand the other person's perspective. The first is based on Janice's experience with her husband bringing home snack foods. The second is based on Jennifer's problem with her mother commenting on other people's weight and appearance.

Example 1: Trying to understand her husband's perspective, Janice started by saying, "I know that you enjoy eating snack foods at night when we watch TV…"

Example 2: Jennifer was quite frustrated with her mother, especially because she felt that her mother's concern with appearances had contributed to Jennifer's own anxiety with weight and shape. However, in trying to understand her mother's emphasis on appearances, she realized that her mother was someone who was always aware of appearances—whether it was a person's appearance, the decorating of a room, or the beauty of the scenery. Jennifer decided to start with this: "I know that you are a very observant person and you notice what people look like . . ."

Now you try it. Do your best to think about where the other person is coming from, and express this in as neutral a manner as possible:

*I know that...*_____

Step 2: Describe what the other person has been doing that is causing you a problem. You must do this in neutral, factual terms. Watch that there is no sting in what you say.

Example 1: Janice tried very hard to stick to the facts in describing what would typically happen in the evening: "When you open up the chips and offer me some..." She did not say, for example, "When you don't even think about me and you offer me that junk food..."

Example 2: Jennifer also tried to stick to a neutral description of her mother's behavior, even though she was tempted to throw in a sting: "When you tell me what you think of other people's weight or appearance..." She did not say, for example, "When all you ever do is comment on people's weight or appearance..."

Now you try. Remember to just describe what happens in as neutral and factual a manner as possible:

*When you . . .*_____

Step 3: Now describe how the behavior in step 2 makes you feel and why. Keep it personal; start with "I feel."

Example 1: Janice concluded her description of her own reaction to her husband's behavior by saying, "I feel afraid that I'm going to fall off my plan, because the chips are too big a temptation for me."

Example 2: Jennifer found it quite easy to explain how her mother's behavior made her feel: "I feel anxious that you and everyone else are thinking about my weight and are critical of my appearance."

Now you try. Describe both the emotion you feel (for example, "afraid" or "anxious") and why you feel this way:

*I feel . . .*_____

Step 4: Now ask for what you want. Keep it simple. If you don't have a particular solution in mind, suggest that both of you try to solve the problems together.

Example 1: Janice didn't want her husband to feel that she was telling him what to do, and she didn't really have a solution she felt comfortable with either. She decided to see if they could solve the problem together: "I'm not exactly sure how to solve this problem, because I want you to enjoy your evening. Would you be willing to join me in a healthier snack? Or do you have another idea?"

Example 2: Jennifer knew what she wanted. She wanted her mother to stop making comments about people's appearances when she was around. She decided to keep her request simple: "I would really appreciate it if you tried not to comment on other people's appearances when you are with me."

Now you try.

I… _____

If you put it all together, you have your complete assertiveness script. Here are Janice's and Jennifer's assertiveness scripts:

"I know that you enjoy eating snack foods at night when we watch TV. When you open up the chips and offer me some, I feel afraid that I'll fall off my plan, because the chips are too big a temptation for me. I'm not exactly sure how to solve this problem, because I want you to enjoy your evening. Would you be willing to join me in a healthier snack? Or do you have another idea?"

"I know that you are a very observant person and that you notice what people look like. When you tell me what you think of other people's weight or appearance, I feel anxious that you and everyone else are thinking about my weight and are critical of my appearance. I would really appreciate it if you tried not to comment on other people's appearances when you are with me."

Try putting your whole script together:

_____

_____

_____

_____

_____

_____

The script, if created according to the steps above, will be respectful of the other person due to your effort to understand the person's perspective and choose neutral and factual language. It should also allow you to communicate your needs effectively. Whatever the outcome, you can feel good about yourself.

WHAT IF THE OTHER PERSON BECOMES DEFENSIVE?

It's always difficult to hear that you have done something that has upset someone. Sometimes, no matter how tactful and gentle your attempts to communicate are, the other person will respond defensively to the suggestion that he has done anything wrong. So what can you do?

Be Patient and Appreciative. Sometimes the person communicates his defensiveness through his manner more than through what he says. For example, Janice's husband might stand up, take the chips, and roughly throw the bags into the cupboard. Jennifer's mother, in a huffy tone, might say, "Fine," but refuse to go on with the conversation. In both these situations, the person may actually understand the point you are making but simply need time to get over the shame and anger at being corrected. In these situations, it may be helpful to give the person the time she needs. Later, thank the person for listening and for being willing to help—even if you don't think her attitude was helpful.

"Honey, thanks for putting the chips away tonight. I know that wasn't your preference. I really appreciate your supporting me in the changes I'm making."

"Mom, thanks for listening to me about the weight thing; I really appreciate your helping me work at being more self-accepting."

Actively Listen and Repeat the Request. Sometimes, however, the person reacts defensively by fighting back and accusing you. This is much harder to deal with. If you have a short fuse, you might explode into anger yourself, and soon both of you are yelling—exactly the situation you were trying to avoid. Or, if you rarely speak up for yourself, you may find yourself apologizing and backing down, angrily regretting your efforts to express your needs. Neither of these options needs to be the outcome if you can keep your cool and simply acknowledge what the person is saying. You don't need to agree; you just need to make it clear that you are trying to understand the other person's perspective. This is often called "active listening."

Janice's husband:	"Well, it's not like I'm the only one bringing snack food home. And you don't need to say yes when I offer you food. I'm only being polite. You have to show some self-control!"
Janice:	(in a neutral tone) "So, from your point of view, you are trying to be polite, and it's up to me to control myself."
Janice's husband:	"Yeah, exactly! Just because you are on some diet doesn't mean that the rest of us have to change our habits!"
Janice:	(actively listening again) "So you don't think I should impose on you just because I'm changing things for myself."
Janice's husband:	"Yes, exactly."
Janice:	(acknowledging his perspective and repeating her request) "Okay, I hear that you think it's up to me to manage my eating. I would still appreciate your support, and I'm wondering if we could come up with a solution together."

Now that her husband has made his point and feels Janice has heard him, he's better able to help solve the problem, even though his attitude might not be perfect. She knows that if she stays calm, he's likely to become less defensive as they talk.

Notice that when you engage in active listening, you don't agree or disagree, and you don't approve or disapprove of what the other person is saying. You simply check out that you have understood what the person is saying. Try starting with phrases like "So you are saying . . ." or "So you feel . . ." or "Just to be sure I understand, you want . . . ." If you have misunderstood, you will be corrected. If you got it right, the person will agree and perhaps go on to elaborate. Once he has had his say, acknowledge that you have heard him and come back to your original request.

Try responding in an active listening way to Jennifer's mother, who has responded defensively:

Jennifer's mother: (in a hurt tone) "Well, that's fine. I just can't seem to do anything right in your eyes. I just won't say anything anymore."

What might you say if you were actively listening? Write it out below:

_____

_____

_____

There are many ways you might respond that would involve actively listening. You might try saying, "So you feel that you can't do or say anything right around me." It wouldn't be active listening if you attempted to reassure her by saying, "Mom, of course, you do things right; please don't be mad." It would also not be active listening if you disagreed with her, saying, "Mom, I never said that; I just asked you to not comment on other people's weight." Nor would it be active listening if you were sarcastic or disrespectful: "Yeah, right Mom, you are *always* doing things wrong." Try out your active listening skills in everyday conversation. Active listening is especially helpful when the person you are listening to feels upset at you or someone else.

CHOOSING THE RIGHT TIME TO SPEAK YOUR MIND

If you have trouble being assertive, you may think you will wait until you feel upset with the person, so your anger can give you the courage to speak your mind. If you have carefully prepared your script, this might work out fine. However, there are pitfalls with this approach:

- If you feel angry or upset, it may be difficult for you to manage your tone of voice or to respond effectively if the other person becomes defensive.

- You don't have a chance to gauge the other person's mood. If the other person is tired or irritable, your talk isn't as likely to go smoothly. Ideally, you would choose a time when the other person is likely to be receptive.

- You won't have as much control over the timing of your talk. You might end up unable to resolve the issue, because one of you may have another commitment.

- You won't have control over the location of your talk. Ideally, you may wish to have privacy. You may find yourself in a public setting trying to manage a potentially emotional conversation.

For these reasons, we suggest that you take the initiative and choose an advantageous time and location.

Where and when would you choose to speak to the person you have identified? When is this person likely to be in a receptive mood?

_____

_____

_____

ASSERTING YOUR RIGHTS MORE BROADLY

Are you a larger person who feels inspired by this book or other life experiences to advocate for size acceptance more broadly than in your personal world? If so, there are others who feel the same way. You may want to reinforce your own efforts toward size acceptance by communicating or working with people who share the same knowledge, understanding, and life experiences. There are many websites and organizations promoting size acceptance. For a current list, do an Internet search for "Largely Positive," or write to Largely Positive Inc., P.O. Box 170223, Glendale, WI 53217, USA. You can also check out the Obesity Action Coalition at www.obesityaction.org.

You may want to write e-mail, send letters, or call companies or the media when you see or hear something about weight and shape that you feel is wrong or potentially harmful. Not only might you contribute to social change, but your sense of self-worth will also be strengthened and you will be a wonderful role model for others around you.

CHAPTER CHECKLIST

You have successfully completed this chapter when:

O   You have identified problematic relationships in your life.

O   You have identified what gets in the way of your being assertive.

O   You have looked at both indirect (hinting) and direct (assertiveness) methods for communicating your needs.

O   You have written out at least one assertiveness script to deal with your interpersonal problem.

O   You have practiced active listening as a method for dealing with defensiveness.

O   You have considered ideal circumstances for delivering your assertiveness script to the person you have in mind.

O   If you are interested, you have begun to explore ways to more broadly assert your rights and fight against size- and weight-based discrimination.

What do you do next, and when?

O   This is the last of the chapters devoted to overcoming the obstacles in the way of your following your eating and activity plan. Continue working on these obstacles until you feel that your eating and activity plan is going relatively smoothly. This can take up to six months.

O   Once you feel that your lifestyle plan is going well, you may wish to address your body image concerns by working through chapters 10 and 11.

CHAPTER 10

Enhancing Your Well-Being: Dealing with Body Dissatisfaction

Chances are that your main reason for picking up this book was to feel better about your body. You are not alone. Wanting to feel more physically attractive is the most common reason given by women, and a significant minority of men, for wanting to lose weight (Levy and Heaton 1993). We want you to feel good about your body but also see body satisfaction as something you strive for, independent of your body weight. Whether you've chosen to work at healthy living or at weight loss, the strategies in this chapter and the next offer you useful ways to work at feeling good about yourself.

HOW TO USE THIS CHAPTER

Changing the way you feel about your body will not happen instantly. You can't tackle every aspect of your body dissatisfaction at once, so the text in this chapter and the next is organized so that you can do the work one week at a time. If you are serious about feeling better about your body, don't just read the chapters; make sure that you actually do the tasks assigned for the week. You will be impressed at how your hard work pays off!

We would suggest that you give yourself at least eight weeks to practice implementing your eating and activity plan before starting to work on this chapter. You may even want to give yourself a good six months of following your plan and working through challenges before starting to work on body image. If you feel impatient to start, remember that you are trying to make changes that will last a lifetime. Take the time to do it right.

WHAT'S YOUR GOAL IN TRYING TO IMPROVE YOUR BODY IMAGE?

The goal in working on body satisfaction is to achieve something quite different from the perfect body. You are working to accept yourself, even though you recognize that your appearance may be less than ideal. Good body image means that there are some aspects of your appearance that you like, there are some aspects of your appearance that you tolerate, and most of the time you aren't thinking about your appearance at all because you are focused on the meaningful and important things in your life. This is what you are aiming for.

WEEK 1: THE BRIDGE FROM LIFESTYLE TO BODY SATISFACTION

We want you to consider your beliefs about weight and weight control. It turns out that your beliefs about weight control are strongly related to how you feel about your body. Before continuing, complete the following questionnaire:

Weight Control Beliefs Questionnaire

Please read each statement and decide how well each statement describes your beliefs:

If the statement is *not true* of your beliefs, circle NT.

If the statement is *slightly true* of your beliefs, circle ST.

If the statement is *moderately true* of your beliefs, circle MT.

If the statement is *very true* of your beliefs, circle VT.

Be sure to respond to every statement.

1. I believe I should control my weight.   NT   ST   MT   VT

2. I try to live a healthy lifestyle and let my weight go to what is natural for me.   NT   ST   MT   VT

3. I focus on healthy living rather than on controlling my weight.   NT   ST   MT   VT

4. If I work at it, I should be able to keep my weight where I want it.   NT   ST   MT   VT

5. I try to accept the weight that is natural for me and focus on living a healthy lifestyle.   NT   ST   MT   VT

6. If I stick to the right exercise and eating plan, I should be able to achieve the weight and shape I want.   NT   ST   MT   VT

7. If I am living a healthy lifestyle, my body is likely at the weight I am meant to be.   NT   ST   MT   VT

145

8. It is important to me that I accept the weight that comes with living a healthy lifestyle.		NT ST MT VT
9. The main thing that determines my weight is what I myself do.		NT ST MT VT
10. If I am careful, I can control my weight.		NT ST MT VT
11. I'd rather live healthily and accept that we all come in different shapes and sizes.		NT ST MT VT
12. If my weight is more than I want it to be, then I am at fault.		NT ST MT VT
13. Whether I gain, lose, or maintain my weight is within my control.		NT ST MT VT
14. I am comfortable letting my weight fluctuate naturally.		NT ST MT VT
15. I focus on healthy eating rather than trying to control my weight.		NT ST MT VT
16. If I want to be a certain weight, I can make it happen.		NT ST MT VT
17. I focus on healthy exercise rather than trying to control my weight.		NT ST MT VT

Note: Reprinted with kind permission from Springer Science and Business Media, Laliberte, Newton, McCabe, and Mills, 2007, 867–68.

Scoring Your Questionnaire

The Weight Control Beliefs Questionnaire has only been studied in women, so the information provided below is more applicable to you if you are a woman. If you are a man, you can calculate your scores and compare them to the ranges given below, but we are less certain that they apply in exactly the same manner.

For all statements, score NT (not true) as 1, ST (slightly true) as 2, MT (moderately true) as 3, and VT (very true) as 4. You might want to put your score for each statement beside its number on the left-hand side of the table. The item numbers for the statements that measure your belief in controlling your weight (weight control) are listed below. Inside the parentheses below, place your score for each item:

1 (   ) + 4 (   ) + 6 (   ) + 9 (   ) + 10 (   ) + 12 (   ) + 13 (   ) + 16 (   ) =

_____ Weight control score

The item numbers for the statements that measure your belief in striving for a healthy lifestyle and accepting your weight (lifestyle control) are listed below. Inside the parentheses below, place your score for each item as you did for the previous scale:

2 (   ) + 3 (   ) + 5 (   ) + 7 (   ) + 8 (   ) + 11 (   ) + 14 (   ) + 15 (   ) + 17 (   ) =

_____ Lifestyle control score

HOW TO INTERPRET YOUR SCORES

Weight Control Score. When you first began reading this book, you probably believed that weight was something you could and should control. You simply needed to put the necessary effort into controlling your weight and you could reach your goals. This belief is a common one. Research tells us, however, that the more strongly you hold this belief, the more likely you are to be dissatisfied with your body and have poor self-esteem (Laliberte et al. 2007). And, the more strongly you hold this belief, the more likely you are to be a yo-yo dieter and to have had trouble with binge eating (Laliberte et al. 2007; Stotland and Zuroff 1990). If your weight control score falls between 18 and 25, you are like most people in our culture. A score below 18 suggests that you don't really believe that you can and should control your weight; a score in this range is associated with better self-esteem and body satisfaction. If your score falls above 25, you are at a higher risk of being dissatisfied with your body and struggling with your eating.

Lifestyle Control Score. After reading chapter 1, you know that weight is strongly influenced by your biology. You may have decided to focus on maintaining a healthy lifestyle and accepting that your body would regulate your weight. Research shows that this belief in striving for a healthy lifestyle and allowing your body to do what's natural for you is strongly related to feeling satisfied with your body (Laliberte et al. 2007). The stronger this belief, the more likely you are to have better self-esteem and fewer struggles with eating. If your lifestyle control score falls between 20 and 27, you are like most people in our culture. If your score falls above 27, you are very likely to have good body satisfaction. If your score falls below 20, you are likely to feel dissatisfied with your body and have greater struggles with eating.

There's nothing wrong with improving your appearance. However, to have lasting satisfaction, you need to have a healthy balance between your willingness to work at self-improvement and your willingness to accept your biological limits and work with realistic expectations.

What if I Chose the Healthy Living Option?

The belief in striving for a healthy lifestyle and accepting the weight that results from it is very consistent with the healthy living option recommended in this book. If you chose this option, you have planned your eating and activity to meet your body's needs and you have allowed your body to find its "natural" weight. Your "natural" weight will have been influenced both by what you have inherited genetically and by your eating and activity patterns over your life. If you have maintained a higher weight for a sufficiently long period, your body's "natural" weight may be in the overweight or even obese range, as difficult as it can be to accept this. Regardless of what you weigh, believing in a healthy lifestyle and accepting the weight that results leads to better body satisfaction.

What if I Chose the Weight-Loss Option?

If you chose the weight-loss option, you may be wondering how all this applies to you. After all, aren't you trying to control your weight? Yes, but we think it's important that you also move away from this belief. If you are following the weight-loss option, you have been given very specific eating and activity recommendations. The goal in following these recommendations is that you will experience a reduction in health risks associated with being overweight or obese. The expectation is that you will lose somewhere between 5 and 10 percent of your original weight by following this plan. It would be easy to get completely focused on the amount of weight you are losing, but we want you to try to approach this experience differently. We want you to see your plan as a healthy lifestyle plan chosen for *your* particular needs. You have a lifestyle goal, not a weight goal. Even though you are asked to monitor your weight, this is really to remind you to stick with your plan. You are *not* expected to alter your plan to increase the weight loss; nor are you expected to alter your plan if you find that you are gaining weight. If you gain weight, you are simply encouraged to make certain that you are adhering to your plan. We want your head in the same place as those who have chosen the healthy living option: you are striving for a healthy lifestyle (tailored to your needs) and are working to accept the weight that results from this lifestyle.

What Can You Work on This Week?

☐ If you need to be reminded of the evidence behind the idea that your body regulates your weight, reread chapter 1. Reflect on how it applies to you.

☐ Are you truly following your plan and trying to eat and be active in a healthy manner?

☐ If you find yourself envying others because of their weight, remind yourself that everyone has a natural weight. If you are living a healthy lifestyle, then your body must be the way it is supposed to be.

☐ If you have been counting on activity to make you lose weight, challenge this way of thinking. Emphasize feeling strong, fit, and healthy over losing weight. When you are not expecting or hoping that physical activity will make you lose weight, you can realize that activity is one of the most powerful tools for feeling better in your body.

☐ Come up with ways of improving your appearance that you *know* you can control—things like getting a good haircut, buying clothes that suit you, and making sure nails are well groomed. Make a commitment to your self-care.

Consider the list above and set some specific goals for yourself:

1. _____

2. _____

3. _____

WEEK 2: WHERE DOES YOUR DISSATISFACTION COME FROM?

This week we want you to shake the foundations of your body dissatisfaction. We want you to question what you have learned from your life experiences and the messages you have received from living in a weight-obsessed culture.

Body Dissatisfaction Is *Not* About Your Body

Researchers have found only a weak relationship between body satisfaction and actual objective attractiveness (Feingold 1992). It turns out that what you look like does not completely dictate how you feel about your appearance. This is particularly true when it comes to body weight. There are thin or average-weight people who hate their appearance and think they are too fat, and there are heavy people who feel attractive and contented with their appearance. Give some thought to your own experiences next.

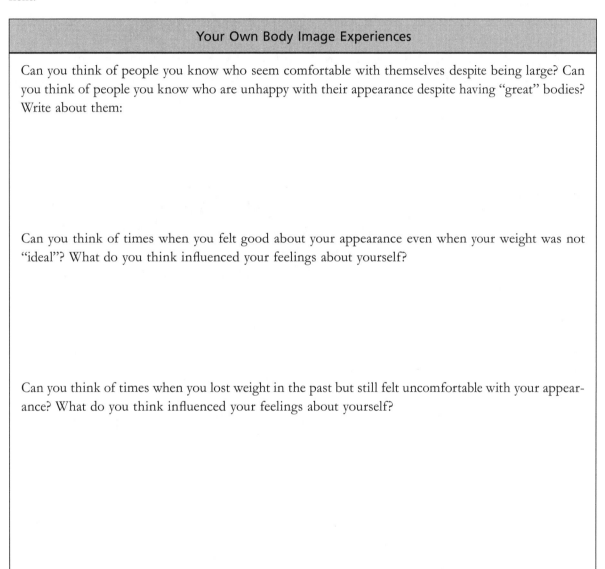

Your Own Body Image Experiences

Can you think of people you know who seem comfortable with themselves despite being large? Can you think of people you know who are unhappy with their appearance despite having "great" bodies? Write about them:

Can you think of times when you felt good about your appearance even when your weight was not "ideal"? What do you think influenced your feelings about yourself?

Can you think of times when you lost weight in the past but still felt uncomfortable with your appearance? What do you think influenced your feelings about yourself?

So what is it that allows some people to feel good in their bodies and leads others to feel so miserable? Your dissatisfaction with your body is not as much about your body as it is about the beliefs you hold about your body.

Is It All in Your Head? Our Toxic Culture and Your Personal History

Your thoughts and feelings about your body didn't appear out of nowhere. Our culture and your own life experiences are key influencing factors.

OUR TOXIC CULTURE

Western culture is very concerned with physical appearance, and weight is held as an important attribute of physical attractiveness. Heavy people aren't just imagining it; they truly face negative evaluation in their social and work lives (Wadden and Stunkard 1985). The media bombards us with messages about the desirability of thinness and the importance of being at an "attractive" weight. Virtually all our celebrities have "ideal" body types, and female celebrities, in particular, are very thin. Our female fashion models are often so thin that they meet criteria for anorexia nervosa. To begin the process of changing your feelings about your body, it's important to evaluate the ways that you expose yourself to our culture's toxic messages. Complete the chart below; note that we have added an example of a response for each item.

Ways You Expose Yourself to Our Culture's Toxic Messages	How You Might Make Healthier Choices
Media (magazines, television, and so on): *I watch make-over shows on TV.*	**Media:** *I will watch a home-decorating show instead.*
People in your life: *My sister is always criticizing her weight.*	**People in your life:** *I will suggest that we make a pact to try to say more positive things about ourselves.*
Places: *My gym has posters of "perfect" people everywhere.*	**Places:** *I will look for a new gym or exercise outside.*

YOUR PERSONAL HISTORY

Even in a culture so focused on the importance of thinness, it's much more likely that you will have learned to dislike your body if you have experienced personal rejection, criticism, or teasing based on your appearance. These experiences can dramatically increase your focus on appearances and increase your body dissatisfaction. Somewhere along the way you may have learned that appearances mattered. We want you to acknowledge these painful experiences but also to begin to fight back and challenge the messages you have received, and may still receive from time to time. Read Karen's chart below and then fill in your own chart to challenge the messages you have received.

Messages I Received	Challenging These Messages
Childhood: *I was a larger child and was teased by the kids at school for being fat.*	*Kids are cruel. When they grow up they often know that what they did was wrong. I was actually just fine as a kid; the kids who teased me were the ones who had the problem.*
Teenage Years: *It seemed like I spent all my high-school years envying the skinny girls; they were beautiful and the boys liked them best.*	*There are always going to be people who are more or less attractive around. High school was probably difficult more because I was so concerned about weight. I actually had friends and even a couple of boys who liked me.*
Young Adult: *I seemed to get so much positive attention when I lost weight. I met my husband and even got a job because of it. Everything fell apart when I gained weight.*	*Although I did get compliments for losing weight, when I think about it, my marriage really fell apart because I was depressed and withdrew from the relationship. My husband always said I looked great. I felt so miserable that I started fights. But not everything fell apart: I got a new job and I still have my son.*
Middle Age: *There are still people in my life telling me that I should lose weight: my family, friends, doctor— even strangers. Clearly I am too big.*	*It would be great if I could wave a wand and lose weight. But I now know that my body is defending this higher weight. I'm living a very healthy lifestyle; for better or worse, this is my body. People really are just uninformed; they think they are helping me when they just don't know what they are talking about.*
Older Age:	

Now you give it a try:

Messages I Received	Challenging These Messages
Childhood:	
Teenage Years:	
Young Adult:	
Middle Age:	
Older Age:	

What Can You Work on This Week?

☐ Catch yourself when you find yourself thinking you would be happier if only you were thinner or more attractive. Challenge these thoughts by reminding yourself that there are people of all shapes and sizes who feel good about themselves. Follow up by getting out there and doing things as if you really did feel good about yourself. Don't wait until your body changes.

☐ Make a commitment to limit your exposure to the message that happiness depends on your appearance or weight loss.

☐ Whenever you find yourself believing that bad things have happened because of your weight, flip this thought around. For example, if people have said something critical or unkind, it teaches you more about them than about you. If something goes wrong in your life, look beyond your appearance to other important factors that may need your attention.

Consider the list above and set some specific goals for yourself:

1. _____

2. _____

3. _____

WEEK 3: GETTING PERSONAL—WHAT YOU SAY TO YOURSELF

This week we want you to take a good look at the things you say to yourself about your body. The exercises below will help you to become more aware of and selective about what you say to yourself.

Mirror, Mirror on the Wall

Look at yourself in a full-length mirror (if you don't have one, then imagine yourself in front of one). Look at your body and allow your mind to do what it usually does. Take note of what you think. What words, phrases, or memories come to mind as you look at your body?

_____

_____

_____

_____

_____

Your Body in Colors

Step 1: Get some crayons, colored pencils, or markers in at least four different colors. In the space below, draw the outline of a body. Don't worry about making it realistic. Color your body parts according to how you feel about them, using a different color for each of the following: positive, neutral, negative, and very negative.

Step 2: For the parts of your body you colored as negative or very negative, write words, phrases, or memories associated with these body parts. Feel free to be as colorful (or as plain) in your language as you have been in your drawing.

Your Drawing and Related Words, Phrases, and Memories

What You Say to Yourself Matters

Imagine letting the following thoughts run unchecked through your head continually: "I'm such a disgusting pig. I am so ugly; look at my fat ass. I have legs like tree trunks. Fat, fat, fat—I am so huge." What impact do you think thoughts like these would have on your mood, your self-esteem, and your willingness to take part in life? One thing's for sure: these kinds of thoughts certainly fuel body dissatisfaction. If we heard someone make these kinds of criticisms to another person, we would be horrified. Yet people who are dissatisfied with their bodies regularly let these kinds of thoughts run unchallenged through their heads.

So What Can You Do About Your Thoughts?

Step 1: Catch yourself thinking these negative, self-critical thoughts.

Step 2: Decide. You can allow your head to go on as it usually does, or you can choose to interrupt this line of thinking.

Step 3: Refocus. What would you think about if you weren't lost in negative thoughts about your body? Would you enjoy the moment (for example, notice the feeling of the water hitting your body in the shower)? Would you think about the day ahead of you? Would you listen more carefully to the person speaking to you? Refocus your thoughts where they belong. It may be a struggle to pull your mind back to where you want it, but it gets easier with time.

FINDING A GENTLER LANGUAGE FOR YOUR BODY

You will also need to find a way of thinking about your body that's at least neutral, and, at best, has positive connotations. In our body-image therapy groups, we ask people to come up with language to describe their bodies. Not all words work well for all people; words that appeal greatly to some are totally wrong for others. Keeping that in mind, here are some words to get you started:

For Women. Soft, feminine, curvy, full-bodied, voluptuous, large, big, "booty-licious," strong, womanly, healthy.

For Men. Stocky, strong, heavyset, big, large, thick, solid, burly, chunky, husky, broad, manly, huggable, meaty.

Feel free to use a thesaurus to find words that work for you. You might also want to think about words that describe the functionality of your body rather than its appearance (such as "efficient," "dependable," "reliable," and "useful"). The idea is to find words that you can relate to and that seem appropriate for your body but have neutral or positive connotations.

Your Body Words

_____

_____

What Can You Work on This Week?

☐ Get a notebook to track your thoughts. Divide each page in half. In the first column, write about the situation in which you caught yourself having negative body-image thoughts. In the second column, write what you did to challenge those thoughts. Did you change your focus, or did you use gentler language for your body? What were your new thoughts? Below is an example:

Negative Body-Image Situation	Challenge
In the mall, shopping for gift. Hating how I look; feeling fat.	_Refocus my thoughts on the gift I need to buy: what would he like? Also, I'm a full-bodied woman._
Getting dressed for work. Nothing fits. Feeling ugly and fat.	_Focus on finding something I know is comfortable. I'm just feeling ugly and fat because my clothes don't fit. Make a note to buy something that fits better. My body is substantial and curvy._

☐ Ask the people in your life for good words. Encourage others to use gentler language when they can.

Consider the list above and set some specific goals for yourself:

1. _____

2. _____

3. _____

WEEK 4: COMPETITIVE COMPARISONS AND MIND READING

If you are dissatisfied with your body, it's very likely that you often find yourself comparing your body to other people's bodies. You may occasionally assume that people are making negative evaluations of your body. Let's consider each of these types of thoughts in turn.

Competitive Comparisons

In our body-image groups we have found that just about everyone owns up to making competitive comparisons—when you compare your body to another person's body. It's interesting to note that most people do not compare themselves to people they believe are less attractive than they are. Rather, people look for the most attractive person in the crowd. Every time you choose to make such a comparison, you reinforce for yourself the importance of appearances; after all, if appearances weren't important, why would you be comparing yourself to others? And, needless to say, the tendency to compare yourself to the most attractive person present is not likely to leave you feeling satisfied with your own body.

Mind Reading

If you think appearance is very important, you likely also believe that *others* think appearance—in particular, your appearance—is very important You may feel that people treat you differently depending on their evaluation of your appearance. In each of these examples, you are "mind reading": assuming that you know what other people are thinking. Mind reading rarely leaves you feeling confident or satisfied with your appearance.

How Do You Challenge Your Thoughts?

You've seen this pattern before. It should be getting familiar by now.

Step 1: Catch yourself.

Step 2: Decide. You can allow your mind to go on as it usually does, or you can choose to interrupt this line of thinking.

Step 3: Challenge your thoughts.

COMPETITIVE COMPARISONS: DEOBJECTIFY

When you objectify someone, that person might as well be a statue, because all that matters is her looks. If you deobjectify someone, you turn that person back into a human being. To deobjectify someone, you have to look that person in the face, or the eyes, and even interact with her. If you can't do this, then try to imagine what that person might be thinking, feeling, or doing in this situation. Commit yourself to only looking at someone if you are actually interacting with that person.

MIND READING: BROADEN YOUR THINKING

When you assume that people evaluate your worth as a person based on your weight, you ignore everything else about yourself that might be important in shaping someone's opinion about you. You ignore their personality, their mood, things that are happening in their lives or in their day—there are so many things that influence another person's behavior and opinion. There are endless things a stranger might be thinking about besides your weight. If you catch yourself mind reading, you need to broaden your thinking and consider that your weight is most likely not even entering the other person's thoughts at all; in fact, the thing that most people are thinking about is themselves!

What Can You Work on This Week?

☐ Notice your negative body-image thoughts and write them in your notebook. Try to identify whether you are *making a competitive comparison* or *mind reading*.

☐ In your notebook, challenge your competitive comparisons (by deobjectifying) and your mind-reading thoughts (by broadening your thinking). See the example below from Jennifer's notebook:

Negative Body-Image Situation	Challenge
Walked across campus and found myself comparing myself to all the best-looking people.	*Tried to deobjectify—I thought about what courses they might be taking. Wondered if they were nervous. Then tried not to look unless talking to the person.*
Store clerk wouldn't acknowledge me. She just kept talking to the other clerk. If I were thin, she wouldn't treat me this way.	*Tried to broaden my thinking. Maybe she is rude to everyone. Maybe she doesn't like her work. Maybe she can't end the conversation easily.*

Consider the list above and set some specific goals for yourself:

1. _____

2. _____

3. _____

WEEK 5: DEALING WITH CLOTHING AND THE MEDIA

Clothing is closely linked to body image. If you are dissatisfied with your body, then every time you try on an item of clothing that doesn't fit right, it can reinforce your dislike of your body. The media is another source of distress for people who feel dissatisfied with their bodies. Even if you avoid watching "toxic" shows on television, you may find it difficult to avoid the influence of media. Just standing in line in the grocery store, you wind up staring at the magazine covers promoting weight loss or showing glamorous pictures of celebrities with "perfect" bodies. So how do you deal with these triggers for body dissatisfaction?

Clothing: The Fitting Room

You are in your favorite clothing store in the mall and see a mannequin dressed in a pair of pants that are just what you are looking for. You find the pants in your size and also grab a couple of other pairs of pants that look appealing. You put on the first pair of pants, and they look nothing like they did on the mannequin. You try on the other two pairs of pants, and one of them looks reasonably good. However, your mood has dropped, and you think to yourself, "I hate my body. I look terrible in most of these clothes—and they are supposed to be my size." You are triggered into experiencing strong body dissatisfaction.

Media: The Perfect Body

It is the evening, and you and your partner are relaxing in front of the television. Your favorite show is about to begin. But first, a commercial comes on, with two fabulously fit and beautiful people—a man and a woman—demonstrating some workout equipment, promising "great" results in very little time. Part of you doesn't really believe it's possible to transform your body into one like the actor's. But another part of you wonders. You think of all the perfect bodies on television and in the magazines, and feel a wave of shame as you think of your body. You wonder if your partner is disappointed in your body, especially in contrast to what's on the television. You feel miserable and depressed for the rest of the evening, and you respond irritably to everything your partner says and does.

How to Change Your Thinking

When dealing with your thoughts, first try to be aware of your emotions. Feelings of shame, embarrassment, sadness, or anxiety are your cues to check in with your thoughts.

Step 1: Catch yourself. You know you feel bad about your body. This is your cue to catch your thoughts.

Step 2: Decide. You can allow your mind to go on as it usually does, or you can choose to interrupt this line of thinking.

Step 3: Challenge your thoughts.

159

CLOTHING: ONE SIZE DOES NOT FIT ALL

If clothing doesn't fit right and you struggle with body dissatisfaction, you will likely blame your body. Here's what you most likely think: "If I had a better body, any clothes I tried on would look great. Clearly the clothes don't look great, so there must be something wrong with my body." This line of thinking seems entirely logical until you think about the many shapes and sizes people of the same height and weight come in: big shoulders, narrow shoulders; large chest, small chest; weight carried around the stomach, weight carried in the thighs and buttocks; thick legs, thin legs; and the list of differences goes on and on. Yet we expect to walk into a clothing store and pick up any item in our size and have it fit beautifully. The many body-shape variations make this very unlikely. Far more likely is that, through a process of trial and error, you will eventually find the clothing cut for your unique body. Before the advent of mass manufacturing, tailors and dressmakers made clothing to suit people's individual shapes and sizes—but now we buy our clothing off the rack.

MEDIA: IT'S HOW THEY MAKE THEIR LIVING

Celebrities are individuals whose careers are built, in part, on their appearance. In order to maintain their appearance, many devote an extraordinary number of hours a day to working out. Female celebrities often survive on a very low calorie diet to keep their weight extremely low. Attractiveness is essential to their livelihood, but not to most of ours. To live a reasonable, balanced life, you wouldn't be expected to work your body as they do. So it's reasonable to accept the looks of celebrities as unrealistic, and somewhat of an aberration. It's impressive, but the lifestyle necessary in order to achieve it isn't realistic or even desirable for most of us.

What Can You Work on This Week?

☐ Try going shopping with a new attitude. Remind yourself that it's inevitable when shopping off the rack to end up with clothes ill designed for your body shape. To increase the likelihood of choosing the right style for your body, check your local bookstore for a book that provides fashion tips for different body types.

☐ Catch yourself when you find that you are comparing your body to those of people in the media. Remind yourself that their living depends on their appearance; it doesn't make sense to compare yourself to them.

☐ Use your body-image notebook to challenge your thinking when you go shopping or when you're exposed to unrealistic body images in the media.

Consider the list above and set some specific goals for yourself:

1. _____

2. _____

3. _____

CHAPTER CHECKLIST

You have successfully completed this chapter when:

○ You have thoughtfully considered your beliefs about weight control. To move toward better body satisfaction, you have tried to focus on your lifestyle and left your weight to your body's biology.

○ You are limiting your exposure to our culture's toxic messages about weight and body image.

○ You have reviewed your personal experiences that contributed to a negative body image and have tried to challenge the messages you received.

○ You have identified negative language that you use for your body and found gentler alternatives. You catch yourself and redirect your attention or challenge your language.

○ You challenge yourself when you catch yourself making competitive comparisons or mind reading.

○ You try to approach shopping and the media with a different attitude.

○ You use your body-image notebook to catch and challenge your thoughts in writing.

What do you do next, and when?

○ Keep working on all the strategies for managing your negative thoughts.

○ If you had life events interrupt your work on body image or you felt you needed to spend longer then one week on some of the material, that's okay. Go at your own pace.

○ Remember to keep following your eating and activity plan!

CHAPTER 11

Changing Behaviors That Support Body Dissatisfaction

In chapter 10, we focused on what was in your head; you worked on becoming aware of your thoughts and managing them, and this work is extremely important in the process of changing your feelings about your body. But it is not enough to stop there. You have to *live* as if you feel satisfied with your body if your feelings about your body are really going to change. In this chapter, you will challenge the behaviors that support body dissatisfaction. This chapter continues the week-by-week approach of chapter 10.

WEEK 6: ELIMINATING CHECKING BEHAVIORS

When you feel dissatisfied with your body or appearance, you might also feel the urge to check your body or appearance. Some checking is normal. But when you struggle with body dissatisfaction, checking often becomes a much bigger problem.

Why Would We Care About Checking?

At first glance, checking seems pretty harmless. For people dissatisfied with their bodies, however, checking can become time consuming and compulsive, and it can lead to a roller coaster of emotion. When you evaluate your reflection in a store window, poke at your stomach, or ask your partner if you look fat, you reinforce your beliefs that your appearance is what defines your worth.

Evaluating Your Checking Behaviors

You may engage in checking in a variety of ways, but the purpose is to evaluate (and hopefully reassure yourself about) your appearance. Take a look at the list below and check off any of the behaviors that you recognize as ones you perform.

Common Checking Behaviors

☐ Weighing yourself

☐ Pinching, pressing, or poking your body parts

☐ Measuring your body or body parts (such as with your hand or a tape measure)

☐ Measuring your body by trying on certain items of clothing

☐ Checking your appearance in mirrors or any reflective surface

☐ Comparing your weight or appearance to others

☐ Asking others if you look fat

☐ Taking pictures of yourself to check your appearance

☐ Trying on different clothing to find the outfit in which you will look your slimmest

☐ Other: _____

On the lines below, write out the checking behaviors that you engage in the most:

_____

_____

_____

Tracking Checking Behaviors

You might be very aware of some of your checking behaviors (for example, weighing yourself). You may be less aware of more subtle checking behaviors that are automatic or routine. Using your notebook (from chapter 10), take at least a couple of days to track your checking behaviors. Take a look at the example from Jennifer's notebook:

Checking Behavior: Mirror/Reflective Surfaces

Time	Describe (size of mirror and what you are looking at)	Triggers (situation, thoughts, emotions)	Body Dissatisfaction (felt better or worse?)
7:15 to 7:30 a.m.	In bathroom, drying hair. Putting on makeup. Face and hair. Small mirror.	Need to see hair and face. Feeling neutral.	Better. Hair looks good today.
7:30 to 8:10 a.m.	At home. Bedroom mirror. Whole body.	Getting dressed. Can't leave mirror, trying on different clothes. Stressed.	Much worse.
9:00 a.m.	At school, going in. Windows and glass door. Whole body.	Want to look okay. There are so many attractive people here. Feeling nervous.	Worse—disappointed.
10:45 to 10:50 a.m.	Washroom at school. Face and body.	Break from class; wanted to check. Bit nervous.	Worse. But hair looks okay.
12:30 to 12:35 p.m.	Washroom at school. Face and body.	Before lunch. Want to check before seeing guys. Anxious.	Worse. More anxious.
12:40 p.m.	Walking into lunchroom, glass door. Whole body.	Nervous.	Much worse. Looked terrible in that door.
1:00 to 1:10 p.m.	Washroom at school. Face and body.	After lunch. Felt so self-conscious today.	Worse. Never look like I hope.
3:30 to 4:00 p.m.	Walking home after classes. Car windows. Face and upper body.	Caught my reflection and then kept looking at myself in all the car windows. Think I look disgusting.	Much worse.
5:00 p.m.	Bathroom at home. Upper body.	Changing into sweats. Don't want to look at myself, but can't resist.	Neutral. Can't tell in sweats that I look so big.
11:00 p.m.	Getting ready for bed. Upper body.	Avoided self until now. Couldn't resist.	Neutral. Wearing pajamas.

As you can see from Jennifer's example, checking rarely made her feel better. It just reinforced what she already felt. She clearly did more checking when she felt anxious about being in situations with other people her age. She actually avoided looking at herself when she no longer needed to be around other people.

Setting Goals for Your Checking Behaviors

Ideally, your goal is to eliminate checking behaviors. For example, after doing the previous tracking exercise, Jennifer decided she wouldn't look at herself in windows or doors anymore. She decided to limit herself to one change of clothing and to only look at herself from the front. During the day, she limited herself to one glance in the mirror (face only) in the bathroom.

As you can see from Jennifer's example, you need to decide what checking behaviors can be eliminated and what checking behaviors need to be limited. You may need to survey some people in your life to get an idea of what limits are reasonable (for example, how much time in front of the mirror in the morning *is* reasonable?).

For each of your checking behaviors, decide on your goals:

1. _____

Goals: _____

2. _____

Goals: _____

3. _____

Goals: _____

4. _____

Goals: _____

5. _____

Goals: _____

Managing Checking in Challenging Situations

If you struggle with body dissatisfaction, there are probably situations that you know are going to make you feel self-conscious and uncomfortable with your body and that are usually accompanied by checking behaviors. One of the most effective ways of making these experiences less distressing is to reduce those checking behaviors. Using Jennifer as an example, she felt very self-conscious about her weight whenever she went out socially. At these social gatherings, she found herself compulsively comparing herself to the attractive women in the group and checking her appearance in every reflective surface she could find. In preparation for a party for a good friend, she made the following plans with respect to her checking:

1. *Only look at people I'm talking to and only look them in the eyes.*

2. *Avoid all reflections, and only check my face and hair briefly when I have to use the bathroom.*

3. *Use one of the strategies from chapter 10: when I catch myself worrying about my looks, I will refocus my attention on what's important, which in this case is chatting with other people or dancing.*

Jennifer successfully implemented her plan (even though at times it felt a little strange) and found that she had a much better time than she usually did. She was actually able to forget about her appearance for a while and enjoy herself.

Can you think of situations that you already know make you feel self-conscious or uncomfortable with your appearance? Write them below:

_____

_____

If one of these situations is coming up soon, come up with a plan for managing your checking:

_____

_____

_____

What Can You Work on This Week?

☐ Track your checking behaviors to find out how often and in what circumstances you are checking your body appearance. Situations that you *know* are going to make you feel self-conscious are most likely to make you check. Plan ahead for these situations if you can.

☐ Set your goals to eliminate or reduce checking behaviors and see if you can begin to implement them immediately.

☐ If you catch yourself checking, don't beat yourself up; just try to stop. Refocus your attention where it would be if you weren't worried about your appearance.

Consider the list above and set some specific goals for yourself:

1. _____

2. _____

3. _____

WEEK 7: AVOIDANCE BEHAVIORS—HOW YOU LIMIT YOUR LIFE

Body dissatisfaction and shame often go hand in hand. Because you dislike your body, or parts of your body, you feel shame at the thought of other people seeing your flaws: your flabby arms, your rolls of fat, or your cellulite. So you try to hide these flaws from view, by covering or camouflaging the parts of your appearance you dislike. Sometimes, you might have hidden yourself entirely, avoiding going out altogether. All of these are examples of avoidance.

Avoidance is not only about hiding your body; it's also about limiting what you do in life because of shame and anxiety about appearances. Jim doesn't coach his children in sports because he feels ashamed of his weight. Karen refuses to go to a spa because of embarrassment, even though this was a great pleasure for her in the past. Jennifer avoids social situations and has refused to buy herself clothing because she feels so ugly. These are all examples of the ways in which avoidance behaviors take the joy out of life.

Evaluating Your Avoidance Behaviors

The following two tables are meant to help you identify your avoidance behaviors. The first table looks at the ways you try to hide your weight or flaws in your appearance. The second table looks at the ways in which you have limited your life in order to keep others from seeing your weight or appearance flaws. In chapter 2 you identified some lifestyle priorities that you avoid because of body-image concerns, so be sure to include these in your table. We have given you examples from the tables that Jennifer, Karen, and Jim filled out, to help prompt you. See if you can fill in *your* avoidance behaviors in the last column.

Ways You Hide Your Body		
Clothing you won't wear	Jennifer: *I'm not buying any new clothes. I specifically won't wear sleeveless shirts, fitted shirts, shorts, or a bathing suit.*	How you avoid:
Clothing you hide behind	Jennifer: *I always wear layers of shirts. I tie a sweater around my waist to hide my bum. I wear baggy clothes. I wear a coat if I can.* Karen: *Big T-shirts and stretch pants.*	How you avoid:
Ways you stand or sit	Jennifer: *When I sit I always lay something across my lap to hide my stomach. I try to sit with my legs up to make my stomach flatter. I suck my stomach in when I stand.*	How you avoid:
Grooming	Karen: *I avoid putting on body lotion, because I don't want to feel my fat.*	How you avoid:
Pictures of yourself	Jennifer: *I always try to be the one taking the picture, and I will delete pictures of me from my friends' cell phones or cameras if I get the chance.*	How you avoid:
Other		How you avoid:

Ways You Limit Your Life Because of Avoidance		
Physical activity	Karen: *I won't go to the gym, because I don't want people seeing how fat I am.* Jim: *I won't do water aerobics because I'm embarrassed to be seen.*	How you avoid:
Eating out or in front of others	Karen: *I only eat diet food in front of others. I don't want people to see the fat lady eating too much.*	How you avoid:
Being touched by others	Jennifer: *I won't let my boyfriend see my body. Lights have to be off. And I don't want him touching my fat, especially my stomach.*	How you avoid:
Places you won't go	Karen: *I won't go to my son's school, the gym, the spa, or the shopping mall.* Jennifer: *I won't go to bars, clubs, or clothing stores.*	How you avoid:
Activities you avoid	Jim: *I won't coach my kids' sports teams.* Jennifer: *I won't go to social events or parties.* Karen: *I won't get a massage.*	How you avoid:

Tracking Your Avoidance Behaviors

You are off to a good start in identifying your avoidance behaviors. Before making changes, however, you will need to spend a week tracking your avoidance behaviors. Using your notebook, create headings as shown in the following table. We have given you an example from Karen's notebook.

Day	Time	Hiding Body	Avoiding Activities
Monday	7:30 a.m.	Didn't use body lotion. Deliberately chose baggiest clothes to wear.	
	8:50 a.m.		I wouldn't drop Brad off in front of the school. Made him walk from corner; I told him it was hard for me to turn the car around.
	9:30 a.m.	Stayed behind the desk when working with clients. Could have sat with them around the coffee table, but wanted to hide.	
	12:30 p.m.		Made an excuse in order to avoid going to lunch with colleagues. Didn't want to be the "fat lady" eating. Ate alone at my desk.
	5:30 p.m.	Wore big loose T-shirt rather than fitted exercise clothes.	Worked out in my basement even though it's a beautiful day and I preferred to walk outside.

What Can You Work On This Week?

☐ Track your avoidance behaviors—both the ways in which you hide your body and the activities you won't take part in because you don't want your body to be seen.

☐ Keep working to eliminate checking, and plan for challenging times.

☐ Continue to catch the thoughts that drive body dissatisfaction, and challenge them.

Consider the list above and set some specific goals for yourself:

1. _____

2. _____

3. _____

WEEK 8: AVOIDANCE BEHAVIORS—PLANNING FOR CHANGE

Now that you have tracked your avoidance behaviors, you may feel overwhelmed by the limitations that shame and anxiety about your body have placed on your life. This week, our goal is to help you eliminate those self-imposed limits by tackling your avoidance behaviors.

Choosing Your Focus

To get started, you will need to choose the avoidance behaviors you will focus on. Of the avoidance behaviors you identified last week, choose those you think need your attention: avoidance behaviors that limit you or interfere with your life in some way.

YOUR LIST OF AVOIDANCE BEHAVIORS

_____

_____

_____

_____

Setting Your Priorities

Now that you have identified the avoidance behaviors you need to work on, you need to decide the order in which you want to work on these behaviors. In general, we would suggest that you start with the behavior that you find the least threatening or least anxiety provoking. We also recommend that you give higher priority to the avoidance behaviors that interfere with your life in some important way. Addressing these behaviors early can alleviate a lot of distress and leave you feeling much better about your life.

Jennifer felt that her avoidance of social events was her most distressing behavior, especially since this often led to conflicts with her boyfriend, Steve. She decided to start with clothing and the ways she hid herself, which seemed an easier task to begin with, and work up to socializing, leaving the scariest for last. Her priorities looked like this:

1. *Clothing*

2. *Hiding (both clothing and the way I stand or sit)*

3. *Intimacy with my boyfriend*

4. *Socializing*

Put your list of avoidance behaviors in order of your priorities:

1. _____

2. _____

3. _____

4. _____

5. _____

Tackling Avoidance: Working from Easiest to Hardest

It's never easy to change behaviors that leave you feeling anxious or ashamed. We are going to develop a *hierarchy* (a plan where you start with easy behaviors and work your way up to the most difficult, until you are doing the things you currently avoid, without anxiety) for each of the avoidance behaviors on your list. You will assign a score to each of the behaviors to reflect how anxious you would feel if you had to engage in the behavior—from 0 (no anxiety at all) to 100 (the worst anxiety you ever felt). Identify the most scary and least scary behaviors first, and then fill in the steps in between. For example:

AVOIDANCE BEHAVIOR: _____*wearing a bathing suit at the beach*_____

Step	Anxiety Level (0 to 100)	Feared Situations
1.	100	Walking in bathing suit at public beach
2.	95	Walking in bathing suit while wearing a wrap at public beach
3.	90	Sitting in bathing suit at public beach
4.	85	Being at pool in bathing suit with male and female friends
5.	80	Being at pool with male and female friends, wearing bathing suit and a wrap
6.	75	Being at pool in bathing suit with female friends
7.	70	Being at pool with female friends wearing bathing suit and a wrap
8.	65	Being at pool in a bathing suit with my family
9.	60	Being at pool with my family wearing bathing suit and a wrap
10.	50	Wearing bathing suit in my house, on my own
11.	45	Wearing bathing suit and shorts with my family
12.	40	Wearing a bathing suit and shorts on my own
13.	35	Wearing T-shirt over bathing suit with my family
14.	30	Wearing a T-shirt over a bathing suit on my own
15.	25	Trying on a bathing suit
16.	20	Hanging a bathing suit where I can see it

As you look at the bathing-suit hierarchy, notice that you may have to break anxiety-provoking behaviors into smaller steps. Ideas for making things harder or easier include thinking about *where* you will engage in the behavior (for example, a public beach versus a private pool), *who* you will be with (for example, people of the same gender are sometimes easier to have around than people of the opposite sex), *when* you will do the behavior (for example, a beach may be more challenging on the weekend than during the week because of who is there), and *how* you will do the behavior (for example, wearing a wrap or not).

Below, we provide you with a blank hierarchy table. Photocopy this, or copy it out in your notebook, and create a hierarchy for each of the avoidance behaviors you identified as your priorities. Don't worry too much if you can't fill in every step; just aim to have at least five to ten steps between the bottom and top of your hierarchy. The scarier the top behavior is to you, the more steps you may need.

AVOIDANCE BEHAVIOR: _____

Step	Anxiety Level (0 to 100)	Feared Situations
1.		
2.		
3.		
4.		
5.		
6.		
7.		
8.		
9.		
10.		
11.		
12.		
13.		
14.		
15.		
16.		

What Can You Work on This Week?

☐ Finish your hierarchies for the avoidance behaviors you prioritized.

☐ Don't try the behaviors on your hierarchy yet! Complete week 9 first.

☐ Keep working on your checking behaviors.

☐ Keep catching and challenging the thoughts that drive body dissatisfaction.

Consider the list above and set some specific goals for yourself:

1. _____

2. _____

3. _____

WEEK 9: AVOIDANCE BEHAVIORS—TAKING BACK YOUR LIFE!

It's time to tackle those avoidance behaviors and take back your life! However, before you start, there are some important things you need to know to make your efforts effective. Remember, your goal is to get over the anxiety and shame you feel at doing the behaviors you currently avoid. For example, we want you to feel comfortable walking on a beach in your bathing suit. The following sections take you through the steps for reducing your anxiety as you work on your hierarchies.

Where Do You Start on Your Hierarchy?

We recommend that you work on one hierarchy at a time. You set your priorities in week 7, so start with the hierarchy you chose then. The goal is to choose a step on the hierarchy that you *know* will make you anxious but that you believe you can manage. You don't want to choose a step that's so overwhelming that you cannot tolerate it and will choose to "escape" it, but you do want a step that will cause some anxiety. So if the step at the bottom of your hierarchy wouldn't cause you any anxiety, then you might want to start with an anxiety level as high as 40 or even 60 on your hierarchy. You *want* to feel anxious—but you also want to feel you can tolerate the anxiety. As you try a step on your hierarchy, you may be surprised to find that you feel much less anxiety than you expected, or you may find that you feel far more anxiety than you anticipated. If this happens, you may need to move things around or create more steps on your hierarchy.

On the line below, write the step on your hierarchy that you think will leave you feeling anxious, but tolerably so:

_____

How Long or How Often Should I Repeat the Behavior?

The key to overcoming anxiety about almost anything is exposure. Exposure means to put yourself in the anxiety-provoking situation long enough or frequently enough that you can experience a reduction in your anxiety or discomfort; this reduction of discomfort helps you learn that you are safe or that it's not as bad as you expected. If you were trying to get over your fear of dogs, the treatment would involve gradually *exposing* you to dogs until you no longer felt afraid. You are going to use this same strategy for overcoming your fear of others seeing your flaws. You are going to expose your body to the world until you are no longer afraid.

When you begin an exposure, rate your anxiety on a scale of 0 to 100 (0 means you feel no anxiety, and 100 means you feel the most anxious you have ever felt in your life). If exposure is going to work, it's important that you stay in the situation or repeat the exposure until your anxiety goes down by half if you can. If this is too difficult, then try to stay in a situation until you feel a smaller drop in your anxiety (for example, from 80 to 60). If you leave or "escape" a situation when your anxiety level is still high, you won't benefit from the exposure and it will still be difficult the next time you encounter the situation. If you begin an exposure—let's say you are wearing a bathing suit while with your family—and you would rate your anxiety at 80 out of 100, then ideally you will stay in that bathing suit until your anxiety drops to 40. Even better would be to stay in the situation until your anxiety goes away.

How Do I Cope While I Do the Exposure?

To make exposure effective, it's really important that you actually *do* the exposure. This means that you have to avoid doing things that help you feel "safe" while doing the exposure. If your goal is to wear a bathing suit at the pool with your friends, you can't stay in the water the whole time or choose a chair that's hidden from view. If you do, then you won't experience a reduction in your anxiety, and you won't learn that you will be okay.

There *are* things you can do to help you cope, however. The most important thing you can do is prepare yourself for how your mind is going to work and what you want your mind to learn. The first step in preparing your mind is to try to anticipate what you will likely think as you begin your exposure. For example, you might expect your mind to think some of the following:

"I look so fat in this bathing suit. They are all going to notice and think I look terrible. They all look so much better in their bathing suits. I feel so uncomfortable."

If you allow your mind to continue like this, you might make it through the afternoon, but you might also remain quite miserable. To make the exposure effective, you might find it useful to be prepared with a different set of thoughts. Use some of the strategies you learned in chapter 10 to help you. An example of more helpful thoughts in this situation might be the following:

Of course I'm going to feel uncomfortable—this is what's supposed to happen in an exposure. Everyone here is wearing a bathing suit, and they don't all have perfect bodies. They like me for who I am and they will accept me even if I don't look perfect. We are here to enjoy each other and the pool; my appearance just isn't the most important thing.

Putting It All Together

You have all the pieces. Now you need to set up your specific exposure plan. The Hierarchy Preparation Plan uses a set of questions to prepare you *each time* you do an exposure. Using this Hierarchy Preparation Plan, you should gradually work your way up the steps of each of your hierarchies. This is going to take some time—it may even take weeks—but if you push yourself to work on your hierarchy every day, you will be amazed at the freedom you feel.

Hierarchy Preparation Plan

1. The hierarchy I am working on: _____

2. The step on the hierarchy I plan to expose myself to: _____

3. How will I make sure I repeat or continue in the situation long enough for my anxiety to go down by about half if possible?

   _____

4. What negative thoughts am I likely to have?

   _____

   _____

5. What thoughts will be more "useful" to me during the exposure?

   _____

   _____

6. My initial anxiety rating (0 to 100) going into the exposure was _____.

7. It took _____ minutes for my anxiety to drop by half or to drop by _____ (other amount).

8. My final anxiety rating (0 to 100) in finishing the exposure was _____.

9. What did I learn from this exposure?

   _____

10. Do I need to repeat this exposure?   Yes [   ]   No [   ]

11. What step in my hierarchy will I work on next?

    _____

12. What impact has the exposure had on my overall comfort with my body?

    _____

What Can You Work on This Week?

☐ Choose a hierarchy and get started. Use the Hierarchy Preparation Plan before each exposure. Work on a step of your hierarchy each day.

☐ Keep working on your checking behaviors.

☐ Keep catching and challenging the thoughts that drive body dissatisfaction.

Consider the list above and set some specific goals for yourself:

1. _____

2. _____

3. _____

WEEK 10: FEELING FAT

If you are dissatisfied with your body because of your weight, you may have days when you struggle with feeling fat—in other words, days where you feel particularly ugly or unattractive. We have given you strategies for catching and challenging your thoughts on these days. We have also urged you to avoid checking behaviors, even on the days when the urge may be stronger. And, in fact, we have pushed you to deliberately engage in behaviors that will no doubt trigger you to feel fat. You have a lot of tools to deal with these difficult times. We want to end your work on body image by challenging you to question the real meaning of "feeling fat."

But What if I *Am* Fat?

Despite what you might think, the experience of feeling fat actually has little to do with your actual body size. People of all sizes walk around feeling at home in their bodies. Even those whose weight interferes with their mobility can experience frustration or fatigue related to their weight, but this is not necessarily what we mean by "feeling fat." Instead, we mean a sense of shame, anxiety, and despair because you believe that your body is unacceptable due to its size or shape. It's a judgment, and it is made by people of every size and shape, even people with nearly "perfect" bodies by today's standards. We recognize that larger people face more messages that reinforce the belief that they should be ashamed of their size. But, regardless of your size, you have every reason to feel good about yourself and the body that's natural for you.

Can You Really *Feel* Fat?

Many of our colleagues, particularly those who work in the area of eating disorders, would argue that you cannot *feel* fat; they would say that you can only *think* you are fat. While this may be technically true, it is not the experience of the clients we work with. Many of them believe that feeling fat isn't simply a thought or evaluation about their size; it's an actual sensation. Regardless of their actual body weight, they claim that they can feel the fat on their bodies; their cells bloated up; and their fat hanging, jiggling, rubbing—even when they are sitting still. This is true for both the smallest and the largest of our clients, and it's related more to their distress than to their body fat. Feeling fat sure feels real, even though it can change from day to day, hour to hour, and minute to minute. The fact that the feeling can change when your body remains the same suggests that, regardless of your size, you need to see the feeling as questionable and wonder why you feel this way today, now.

What Triggers "Feeling Fat"?

There are many experiences in our day-to-day lives that we would all agree might make a person more aware of their weight or size. Take a look at the list below and check off the ones that might trigger you to feel fat:

☐ Seeing your weight go up on the scale

☐ Feeling that your clothes are tighter than they were

☐ Eating a large meal and feeling very full

☐ Being around other people who are talking about their weight or weight loss

☐ Being around other people who you think are very thin or fit and attractive

☐ Hearing someone comment on your weight

☐ Hearing someone comment on someone else's weight

☐ Watching a television show about weight loss or other appearance issues

☐ Reading a magazine article focused on weight loss

☐ Other: _____

Any of the items on the list above clearly focus your attention on your weight. If you already struggle with dissatisfaction, any of these things could trigger you to feel fat.

THE NOT-SO-OBVIOUS TRIGGERS FOR FEELING FAT

The triggers listed above are all fairly obvious triggers; they all pertain directly to weight and shape. For people who struggle with body dissatisfaction, however, there are triggers that are not so obvious.

To explore this, we'd like you to try to answer the following question (without reading ahead): *If it were true that you were as fat, ugly, or unattractive as you feel at your worst, what would it mean about you as a person? What would it say about you? Try to list at least three things:*

_____

_____

_____

This may have been a difficult question to answer. What we are looking for, however, are the qualities you associate with feeling fat or unattractive, even if you are ashamed of these associations.

The attributes you think of on your own are the ones you most powerfully associate with feeling fat. However, if you need help, consider the list below:

- Out of control

- Unlovable

- Lazy

- Failure

- Unlikeable

- Weak

- Unsuccessful

- Worthless

- Other: _____

Although you may associate these attributes with feeling fat, the reality is that these attributes are quite independent of body weight. In fact, these beliefs about yourself can be triggered by many life experiences. For example, when your life is too busy and you feel that you cannot stay on top of things in the way you would like, you may feel "out of control." If you have a fight with your friend, partner, or family member, you can feel "unlikeable" or "unlovable." All of these feelings can be triggered by life events or factors other than your weight, and they can leave you feeling fat. This is because you already connect feeling fat with these attributes.

What Happens When Life Leaves You Feeling Fat?

When life triggers you to feel bad about yourself (for example, to feel unlikeable or as if you're a failure), it can also trigger you to feel fat if the two feelings are connected in your mind. If you struggle with body dissatisfaction, however, the connection between feeling fat and your life may not be obvious at the time. Instead, you may simply feel fat and never stop to question the validity of this feeling. In this case, you are likely to spiral into more negative thoughts about your body, experience an escalation of checking behaviors, and want to avoid being seen. Feeling fat is also likely to leave you much more sensitive to the "obvious" triggers we listed earlier—in other words, you are more likely to feel that your clothes are tighter or to feel sensitive to the remarks others make about their weight and so on.

On the other hand, feeling fat can be a useful signal to you to pay attention to your life. It's not a pleasant signal, but it may have something valuable to tell you. One of our clients described finding herself standing in front of her kitchen sink peeling a carrot and feeling fat. Once she "caught herself" in the feeling, she knew in a flash that she felt this way because she was anxious about starting a new job that evening and doubted she would be liked or successful. Another client, who found herself struggling with the feeling that she was eating too much all the time and that she was fat, was able to recognize that these feelings only became strong whenever her life got too busy and she started falling behind. She had always associated feeling fat with being out of control; in this case her life felt out of control, and she reacted to it by feeling fat. For both these women, the problem was not body weight. The problem was anxiety over other issues. In both these cases, the women benefited far more from addressing the *real* problem than they would have from reacting to feeling fat.

Helping You to Benefit from Feeling Fat

It may be strange to think that there could be an upside to feeling fat when it's such an unpleasant experience. But some of life's most useful signals are unpleasant; for example, pain causes you to attend to something that might injure you, an irritable bowel can let you know that you are under stress, and a cold sore can indicate you need more rest. Feeling fat can be a signal to pull back and consider what's going on in your life. What might be making you feel less sure of yourself in some important way? Once you identify the real issue, you can solve the real problem. You may not immediately stop feeling fat, but the feeling will no doubt disappear as you successfully address the real concerns in your life. In the next week, use your notebook to track the instances in which you feel fat. Note any obvious triggers, but also consider whether life is making you feel unsure of yourself. Then set out to resolve the real issue. See the following example from Jennifer's notebook.

Day	Feeling Fat (describe)	"Obvious" Trigger	Life Trigger	Solution?
Monday	Found myself feeling fat all afternoon.	Had big lunch.	Had argument with Steve on the phone. He's frustrated that I won't go to the party tonight.	I think my feeling fat is because I feel unlikeable. Maybe I should go to the party as an exposure.
Thursday	Felt yucky and fat all day.	Feeling bloated.	Actually, I think it's my period.	Just remind myself it will be over in a few days.
Saturday	Felt fat all morning.	Clothes felt uncomfortable and tight.	I was so hot in the car. I think being hot makes me feel fat.	Challenge thought. Stay cool. Choose clothes that are more comfortable.

Notice that only one of Jennifer's life triggers was related to feeling unsure of herself. She was also able to identify other life triggers that weren't quite as deep but nonetheless left her feeling fat. Look for the significant emotional triggers in your life and then consider lesser factors that might be at play.

What Can You Work on This Week?

☐ Keep track of what happens when you feel fat, and look for both obvious and life triggers. Try to solve the "real" problem. You may still need to manage the situations by catching and challenging your thoughts and keeping your checking behaviors under control.

☐ Keep working on your hierarchies.

☐ Limit those checking behaviors!

☐ Catch and challenge the thoughts that drive body dissatisfaction.

Consider the list above and set some specific goals for yourself:

1. _____

2. _____

3. _____

Weight-Based Self-Esteem: Time for a Change

When you started the process of working on developing a better relationship with your body in chapter 10, it's likely that your self-esteem was strongly tied to your feelings about your weight. In both chapters 10 and 11, we hope that you have begun to untangle your self-esteem from your body image to some extent. As you work on self-acceptance, try to explore aspects of your self-worth and give them more importance than your weight. To do this, you need to reflect on your interests and life more broadly and consider what important factors contribute to your self-esteem. We will prompt you with a list of life areas that contribute to most people's self-worth, but we would like you to try to make the list more personal and specific by identifying your particular strengths or interests under each heading:

FAMILY

Your strengths or interests: _____

_____

FRIENDSHIPS OR SOCIAL LIFE

Your strengths or interests: _____

_____

SCHOOL OR WORK LIFE

Your strengths or interests: _____

_____

ROMANTIC RELATIONSHIP

Your strengths or interests: _____

_____

HOBBIES OR ACTIVITIES

Your strengths or interests: _____

_____

SPIRITUAL LIFE

Your strengths or interests: _____

_____

Good self-esteem results from having many different aspects of your life that contribute to your self-worth. Focusing on only one aspect of yourself (like weight or appearance) as a measure of your worth is to put all your eggs in one basket—and a flimsy basket at that. If your list was lacking in certain areas, give some thought to how you might begin to build each of these areas. It's not that appearance is irrelevant, but it's only *one* part of who you are. We hope that you continue to work on improving your body image and that you also work to develop your sense of self-worth by taking into account the many aspects of who you are.

CHAPTER CHECKLIST

You have successfully completed this chapter when:

○ You have tracked your checking behaviors and set goals to eliminate or reduce them. Keep working on this, particularly when you find yourself struggling with body dissatisfaction. Be vigilant! Don't let checking creep back in.

○ You have created your avoidance hierarchies.

○ You are working on doing your feared activities every day and completing a Hierarchy Preparation Plan for each exposure practice. You may need to repeat some steps until you feel so little anxiety that you know you are ready to move on. Keep working on your hierarchies in the weeks to come. Don't give up until you feel you have overcome your fears!

○ You respond to feeling fat by pulling back to examine both the "obvious" and the "life" triggers that may be playing a role. When you identify life triggers, you set out to solve the real problem. You manage body dissatisfaction by challenging your thoughts, controlling checking behaviors, and *not* backing out of life.

What do you do next, and when?

○ Keep working at all the strategies you have learned—both those introduced in chapter 10 and those described in this chapter.

○ We expect it will take you longer than ten weeks to complete your hierarchies. We also expect that you will have to keep working at all the strategies you have learned if you are to continue to feel better about your body.

○ Continue to chapter 12, where you will plan to maintain your changes over the long term.

Maintaining the Lifestyle Change

We expect it will take at least six months to make the changes suggested in this book before you feel that you have your eating and activity plans well in hand. If you have successfully made changes, then you have worked hard to overcome your personal obstacles and possibly deal with body-image concerns. Take a moment to congratulate yourself for everything you have accomplished. Now take a deep breath and get ready, because the difficult work of maintaining your gains is just beginning.

SUCCEEDING IN THE LONG TERM: WHAT EXACTLY *IS* SUCCESS?

This workbook has asked you to focus on changing your lifestyle. It has emphasized improved health and body satisfaction as the core reasons to make changes to your lifestyle. But how do you know if you are succeeding in your changes? To define success, we can look at three major outcomes across the different weight management options: lifestyle, health, and body image. For each area, you will evaluate your personal strengths and vulnerabilities.

Measuring Success: What the Options Have in Common

No matter what plan you have been following, we can gauge your success by the degree to which you have been able to make changes to your behaviors and your beliefs.

LIFESTYLE

Successful lifestyle change is defined mostly by your ability to follow your plan and change problematic behaviors, not just for a few months but over the long term.

Consider each item below and decide whether it's an area of strength or vulnerability for you.

	Strength	Vulnerability
My eating plan fits easily into my life.	☐	☐
I eat at regular intervals throughout the day.	☐	☐
My eating is balanced across the different food groups.	☐	☐
My activity plan fits easily into my life.	☐	☐
I have chosen physical activity I enjoy.	☐	☐
I can identify triggers when I fall off my plan.	☐	☐
I use strategies to address triggers and get back on track.	☐	☐

HEALTH

For your health, success means that the weight management option you chose has lessened your chronic health problems. All options depend on your lifestyle changes.

Consider the items below and decide if they are strengths or vulnerabilities:

	Strength	Vulnerability
I eat foods high in soluble and insoluble fiber regularly.	☐	☐
I have fatty fish at least twice a week.	☐	☐
I eat more than five servings of fruits and vegetables per day.	☐	☐
I choose orange and dark-green fruits and vegetables often.	☐	☐
I have at least two servings of dairy each day.	☐	☐
I often choose unsaturated fats.	☐	☐
I build thirty to sixty minutes of physical activity into my day.	☐	☐
I am active four to six days per week.	☐	☐
I work with my physician to manage any health concerns.	☐	☐

BODY IMAGE

Success with regard to your body image means that you are increasingly comfortable in your body, and body dissatisfaction no longer interferes with your life. You feel more confident and have skills for dealing with body image issues as they arise. This is an area you will keep working on. Regardless of your weight management choice, good body image depends on your efforts.

Identify your strengths and vulnerabilities below:

	Strength	Vulnerability
I have not relied on weight loss to feel better about myself.	☐	☐
I am focused on healthy lifestyle rather than a weight goal.	☐	☐
I work to catch and challenge negative thoughts.	☐	☐
I resist checking behaviors.	☐	☐
I don't avoid things because of body dissatisfaction.	☐	☐
I look for the deeper reasons behind my "feeling fat."	☐	☐
I know how to deal with people who are hurtful.	☐	☐
I see self-acceptance as the key to good self-image.	☐	☐

Measuring Success: How the Weight Management Plans Differ

Although all the weight management plans have the same fundamental components (as shown in the section above), each plan is suited to different people and is aimed at a different end point. In this section you will evaluate your strengths and vulnerabilities for components that are specific to the weight-management plan you are following.

LIFESTYLE

For the weight management plan you are following, evaluate your progress below.

Healthy Living Plan. Being successful on the healthy living plan means meeting your body's needs, both by eating in a regular and balanced manner and by engaging in regular, moderate physical activity. This plan allows you more flexibility in both your eating and your activity than the various weight-loss alternatives.

Following are items that would describe success on the healthy living plan. Read through the items to identify your personal strengths or vulnerabilities.

	Strength	Vulnerability
I never feel that I'm struggling with hunger.	☐	☐
I feel pleasure from the foods I'm eating.	☐	☐
A couple of times a week I have "exceptional meals."	☐	☐
I informally check my eating for balance from time to time.	☐	☐
I am committed to my activity plan.	☐	☐
I can be flexible with my activity plan when needed.	☐	☐

Weight-Loss Plan (Through Lifestyle Changes, Medication, or Surgery). Being successful on a weight-loss plan requires somewhat different lifestyle changes. Although you are encouraged to stay on your plan whenever possible, you, too, will need to allow for occasional "exceptions"; aim for planned exceptions that differ from your usual plan in their quality (such as a richer choice) rather than the quantity of food. Perhaps the biggest difference between this and the healthy living plan is the need for you to be open to starting over if you regain weight or to considering different weight-management options if your first approach isn't successful.

If you chose a weight-loss plan, consider the items below and whether they represent your strengths or vulnerabilities.

	Strength	Vulnerability
I continue to plan my eating and keep a food diary.	☐	☐
I plan carefully for changes to my routine to stay on plan.	☐	☐
I have adjusted my eating slightly to manage my hunger.	☐	☐
I have allowed for exceptions when I had to.	☐	☐
I prefer fewer food choices, to help me stay on track.	☐	☐
I am active five to six days a week for sixty minutes.	☐	☐
I am willing to start all over again if I need to.	☐	☐
I am willing to research medication if I feel I need it.	☐	☐
I am willing to consider surgery if appropriate.	☐	☐
I would consider the healthy-living option if I couldn't sustain the weight-loss lifestyle and if the other options were not appropriate for me.	☐	☐

HEALTH

Each of the weight-management plans is expected to have a positive impact on your health.

Healthy Living Plan. For the healthy-living plan, the same items you rated in the "Lifestyle" section on page 187 apply here.

Weight-Loss Plan (Through Lifestyle Changes, Medication, or Surgery). Safe weight-loss medications can be helpful tools for individuals who struggle to adhere to lifestyle changes. With this weight-loss option (balanced-deficit diet with or without medication), you have succeeded if you have maintained even 5 percent of your weight loss.

If you chose a weight-loss option, identify your strengths and vulnerabilities below.

	Strength	Vulnerability
I am not frequently losing control of my eating.	☐	☐
I understand that some weight regain is very likely.	☐	☐
I have achieved success if I maintain just 5 percent of my weight loss.	☐	☐
I work closely with my doctor (if I am on medication).	☐	☐
I am closely monitored by my doctor (if I have had surgery).	☐	☐

Weight-Loss Surgery. Weight-loss surgery often reverses significant health risks or health problems related to obesity. You could expect to maintain these benefits as long as you do not have many episodes of "overeating" (remember that overeating after weight-loss surgery may involve an amount much smaller than prior to surgery). This more-invasive option requires adherence to a particular eating pattern, which the surgery helps you maintain, and it can also require the addition of supplements and routine follow-up.

If you chose this intervention, identify your strengths and vulnerabilities below.

	Strength	Vulnerability
I am not frequently losing control over my eating.	☐	☐
I avoid foods that can pose problems.	☐	☐
I take the required supplements.	☐	☐
I am closely monitored by my doctor.	☐	☐

BODY IMAGE

For the weight management plan you are following, evaluate your progress next.

Healthy Living Plan. If you have chosen the healthy living plan, then you are aiming for self-acceptance as a strategy for body satisfaction, and you expect your body to remain relatively stable over time.

Identify your strengths and vulnerabilities below.

	Strength	Vulnerability
I am no longer trying to change my weight.	☐	☐
I am trying to accept my "natural" weight.	☐	☐

Weight-Loss Plan (Through Lifestyle Changes, Medication, or Surgery). If you chose any of the weight-loss options, you have also been encouraged to work at self-acceptance, but it may be more difficult not to get invested in the weight loss as your means of feeling better about yourself. Success in the long term will depend on your ability to accept yourself regardless of changes in your weight.

Identify your strengths and vulnerabilities below.

	Strength	Vulnerability
I try to accept whatever weight change results from my plan.	☐	☐
I do not make my plan stricter to manipulate my weight.	☐	☐
I try to rely on self-acceptance rather than weight loss.	☐	☐
I am prepared to work at accepting myself if I gain weight.	☐	☐

AN OVERVIEW AND PLAN FOR DEALING WITH YOUR VULNERABILITIES

We hope you have identified areas of strength in your weight-management efforts. If you have found vulnerabilities, it's important that you focus on these areas. The previous items are based on various chapters in the book—planning, dealing with obstacles, and addressing body-image concerns—so once you have identified your areas of vulnerability, locate and review the appropriate sections. Make a commitment to continue to review these sections until you can confidently check them off as strengths, rather than vulnerabilities.

Your vulnerabilities:

_____

_____

_____

_____

Parts of book you intend to review:

_____

_____

_____

_____

Weight Loss: Special Risk of Relapse

The first six to twelve months after you have successfully lost weight appears to be a time of increased vulnerability, due to an unfortunate combination of biological and environmental factors. At around six months, weight loss tends to plateau. Your body engages various biological defenses to prevent further weight loss. You also develop a heightened sensitivity to tasty foods at around this time. Your relapse risk may be further increased by your feeling a bit discouraged at having to maintain the restrictions of your lifestyle without experiencing the payoff of further weight loss. It may be even harder to continue, in the face of the small weight regain that will almost inevitably occur. If you aren't prepared for all this, you are likely to throw in the towel at that point. Although medication and surgery can help, these options are not for everyone. We want to help you to maintain your success. To do this, let's take a look at the factors found to enhance the maintenance of weight loss:

1. Have a weight-loss professional to talk with when you have a setback. During difficult times, checking in with a dietitian, physician, psychologist, or other health care professional with weight-loss experience is more likely to keep you on track.

2. Participate in a weight-loss support group. If there are different options available in your area, interview the facilitators first to be certain that their approach is compatible with your goals. People in these groups can offer invaluable support and advice during difficult times, so be sure to admit when you are faltering, and pick their brains for possible solutions.

3. Include your friends and family. If the people closest to you can attend your support-group session, you are more likely to successfully stay on track.

4. Regular exercise seems to be a key ingredient in keeping people on track. It's also extremely important that the exercise be convenient—preferably something you can do at home. For example, a treadmill may be a good investment if you can afford to buy one. Convenient, at-home exercise has been found to be even better than having a personal trainer in making it more likely that you will maintain your weight loss. Exercise done in smaller intervals of time was just as effective as one long bout of exercise (Jakicic, Wings and Winters 1999).

5. Limit your food choices. Some of the most successful weight losers are those who adhere to eating plans with less variety. More options seem to increase the likelihood that you will fall off your plan.

If you are committed to maintaining a significant percentage of your original weight loss (and notice that we still expect some weight regain), can you put any or all of the above strategies into place? Next brainstorm how you would do this and see if you can commit to a particular solution. Use those problem-solving skills you learned in chapter 7.

1. Finding professional support

   Your brainstorming ideas: _____

   _____

_____

Which will you try? _____

2. Joining a support group

   Your brainstorming ideas: _____

   _____

   _____

   Which will you try? _____

3. Involving friends and family in the plan

   Your brainstorming ideas: _____

   _____

   _____

   Which will you try? _____

4. Exercising in a convenient way

   Your brainstorming ideas: _____

   _____

   _____

   Which will you try? _____

5. Limiting your food choices

   Your brainstorming ideas: _____

   _____

   _____

   Which will you try? _____

Weight Loss: What If You Really Do "Fall off the Wagon"?

Although we have been focusing on how to stay on track, there's always a possibility that you will fall back into your old habits. We often say to our patients that wellness or success doesn't happen because you do everything right; it comes because you are persistent and keep working to solve problems that arise. Sometimes, however, life and circumstances combine to create problems and distractions, and despite your best intentions, the work you've done begins to slip away on you. So, if you regain some or all of your weight, what are your choices?

1. **You can decide to give up.** This is always an option. You can just go back to the lifestyle you had before you decided to make changes. In some ways this is the easiest choice, but it's also the most disheartening. You chose to work for change for reasons you outlined in chapter 2. If you feel like giving up, we encourage you to read that chapter again and decide if you still have reasons for changing.

2. **You can try again.** Try to understand that you have not "failed"; your biology has simply overcome your efforts, at least temporarily. Your body's pressure to return to your "natural" weight is relentless. So be gentle with yourself. When you feel strong enough and when you feel your life is stable enough, you can begin the process followed by many successful weight losers, and try again. Persistence is the key! If you decide to try again, you may wish to bring in reinforcements. You may decide that you need to speak to your physician about medication options to help you deal with these biological pressures. If your weight is high enough, you may want to consider weight-loss surgery.

3. **Change strategies.** If you have lost and regained weight before, you may decide that you are tired of the weight-loss–weight-regain treadmill. You may feel that you've tried all the approaches you can think of. Remember that you *do* have another option. You could try the healthy living approach to weight management. It's hard to give up on the dream of weight loss, especially if you have pursued it for many years. But giving up on weight loss doesn't mean you have to give up on improved health or better body image. If you are considering the healthy living option, go back to chapters 3 and 4 to modify your plan.

Janice successfully maintained her weight loss for many years. She lost nearly forty pounds and maintained this loss through careful eating and regular, intense activity (she alternated between running, speed walking, and taking spinning classes). One winter, her life just became ridiculously busy: she found herself swamped with her children's extracurricular activities and her demanding work life. Her activity dropped off and she relaxed her eating habits. She regained twenty-five pounds. She felt surprised and reassured when she was told she was still a successful weight loser, because she thought regaining most of her weight would have defined her as unsuccessful. She wasn't discouraged by the weight regain, because she also knew that she could be successful for long periods. She decided to begin the weight-loss process again. She knew that she needed to figure out how to balance her time better so that she could take care of her needs again. She did some problem solving and has gotten back on her plan. She's in no hurry, because she sees weight management as a long-term commitment. She just focuses on staying with her plan and managing problems as they come up.

Dealing With High-Risk Situations

Regardless of the weight management plan you have chosen, you may encounter certain high-risk situations that could put anyone at risk for falling off plan. If you are following the healthy living plan, you have more flexibility, in that you can consider some of these events "exceptional" meals, of which you are allowed two per week. Some situations, however, push even these limits, so we want you to think ahead for the next week, month, or even year to see if you will be facing any of these high-risk situations. Check off the ones you see in your present or future:

Here are some of those common high-risk situations:

■ Holidays, especially those that revolve around food

■ Special occasions (weddings, baby showers, birthday parties)

■ Travel (cruise ships, family vacations)

■ Work dinners and lunches

■ Business travel and hotel stays

■ Eating out, especially at buffets

■ Times of stress

■ Events that involve alcohol

■ A work environment where food is constantly available

■ Shift work

Reviewing Your Own History: Finding the High-Risk Situations

Although we have listed some of the common high-risk situations above, the most important information for you will come from your own past experiences. Take a moment to think back over your dieting history. If you have tried to lose weight or eat healthily and be active in the past but got off track, what do you think went wrong? What can you learn from your past dieting or healthy-eating attempts that could help you stay on track this time? Give some thought to high-risk situations, high-risk emotions, or high-risk interactions that derailed your efforts in the past. For each high-risk situation you recall, fill in one of the following boxes.

Situation: _____

Why is this situation a challenge for you? _____

What have you tried in the past? _____

How successful has this solution been? _____

_____

Situation: _____

Why is this situation a challenge for you? _____

What have you tried in the past? _____

How successful has this solution been? _____

_____

Situation: _____

Why is this situation a challenge for you? _____

What have you tried in the past? _____

How successful has this solution been? _____

_____

In chapter 7, you were introduced to the strategy of planning ahead and problem solving. This technique can also be applied when you are dealing with risky situations as you move into your long-term efforts. If you identified emotions or interpersonal problems as triggers for relapse, then you might need to use some of the strategies you learned in chapter 8 for emotional triggers or chapter 9 for interpersonal triggers. Use the Problem-Solving and Planning-Ahead Worksheet from chapter 7 to address each high-risk situation you identified above.

YOUR JOURNEY ISN'T OVER—IT'S JUST BEGINNING

Having made it to this point, you deserve to be congratulated for your hard work and effort. Although you have reached the end of this book, you are now embarking on a journey of maintaining the changes you have made. Do not leave this book on a shelf to gather dust; use it frequently, because it will be a valuable tool in your efforts to keep on track with your lifestyle goals. As obstacles come up or as motivation wanes, pick up the book and turn to the relevant chapter. Review your worksheets, increase your awareness, and give yourself some strategies to manage the obstacles that arise on your path.

CHAPTER CHECKLIST

You have successfully completed this chapter when:

O You have identified what makes you vulnerable to falling off your weight-management plan and decided what chapters in this workbook you need to review.

O If you are following a weight-loss plan, you understand the risk for relapse and you are familiar with the factors that seem important in helping people to maintain their weight loss. You have a plan for incorporating these strategies into your life.

O You have thought through the common high-risk situations for falling off your plan (your workplace, your schedule, your social life) and looked at factors that contributed to past difficulties with staying on your plan. You have solved problems around these high-risk situations and feel you have a good plan for managing them successfully.

What do you do next, and when?

O Continue to use the techniques you have learned in the book to help maintain your weight-management plan, hopefully for years to come.

O If you run into difficulties, get the support you need to get back on track.

O Keep looking for high-risk situations and keep learning from your mistakes. Keep seeing setbacks as opportunities to learn more about yourself.

O If you truly fall off your plan, try to be gentle with yourself. When you are ready, consider your options again, and learn from your experiences.

O Enjoy your new relationship with your body and with food!

References

Allison, D. B., R. Zannolli, M. S. Fatih, M. Heo, A. Pietrobelli, T. B. VanItallie, F. X. Pi-Sunyer, and S. B. Heymsfield. 1999. Weight loss increases and fat loss decreases all-cause mortality rate: Results from two independent cohort studies. *International Journal of Obesity* 23(6):603–11.

American Psychiatric Association. 2000. *Diagnostic and Statistical Manual of Mental Disorders (DSM-IV-TR)*. 4th ed. Washington, DC: American Psychiatric Association.

Barlow, C. E., H. W. Kohl III, L. W. Gibbons, and S. N. Blair. 1995. Physical fitness, mortality, and obesity. *International Journal of Obesity* 19(Suppl. 4):S41–44.

Bouchard, C., A. Tremblay, J. P. Despres, A. Nadeau, P. J. Lupien, G. Theriault, J. Dussault, S. Moorjani, S. Pinault, and G. Fournier. 1990. The response to long-term overfeeding in identical twins. *New England Journal of Medicine* 322:1477–82.

Campbell-Sills, L., D. H. Barlow, T. A. Brown, and S. G. Hoffman. 2006. Acceptability and suppression of negative emotion in anxiety and mood disorders. *Emotion* 6:587–95.

Corbett S. W., J. S. Stern, and R. E. Keesey. 1986. Energy expenditure in rats with diet-induced obesity. *American Journal of Clinical Nutrition* 44:173–80.

DiClemente, C. C., and M. M. Velasquez. 2002. Motivational interviewing and the stages of change. In *Motivational interviewing: Preparing people for change,* ed. W. R. Miller and S. Rollnick. New York: Guilford Press.

Fabricatore, A. N., C. E. Crerand, T. A. Wadden, D. B. Sarwer, and J. L. Krasucki. 2006. How do mental health professionals evaluate candidates for bariatric surgery? Survey results. *Obesity Surgery* 16:567–73

Feingold, A. 1992. Good-looking people are not what we think. *Psychological Bulletin* 111:304–41.

Fontaine, K. R., M. S. Faith, D. B. Allison, and L. J. Cheskin. 1998. Body weight and health care among women in the general population. *Archives of Family Medicine* 7:381–84.

Food and Nutrition Board, National Research Council. 1989. *Diet and Health: Implications for Reducing Chronic Disease Risk.* Washington, DC: National Academy Press.

Foreyt, J. P., G. K. Goodrick, R. S. Reeves, and A. S. Raynaud. 1993. Response of free-living adults to behavioral treatment of obesity: Attrition and compliance to exercise. *Behavior Therapy* 24:659–69.

Foster, G. D. 2006. Clinical implications for the treatment of obesity. *Obesity* 14(Suppl. 4):S182–S185

Foster, G. D., T. A. Wadden, and R. A. Vogt. 1997. Body image before, during, and after weight loss treatment. *Health Psychology* 16:226–29.

Foster, G. D., T. A. Wadden, R. A. Vogt, and G. Brewer. 1997. What is a reasonable weight loss? Patients' expectations and evaluations of obesity treatment outcomes. *Journal of Consulting and Clinical Psychology* 65(1):79–85.

Gleeson, M. 2007. Immune function in sport and exercise. *Journal of Applied Physiology* 103:693–99.

Gregg, E. W., and D. F. Williamson. 2002. The relationship of intentional weight loss to disease incidence and mortality. In *Handbook of obesity treatment,* ed. T. A. Wadden and A. J. Stunkard. New York: Guilford Press.

Gross, J. J. 1998. The emerging field of emotion regulation: An integrative review. *Review of General Psychology* 2:271–99.

Harris, J., and F. Benedict. 1918. A biometric study of human basal metabolism. *Proceedings of the National Academy of Sciences US* 12:370–73.

Hayes, S. C., K. Strosahl, and K. G. Wilson. 1999. *Acceptance and Commitment Therapy: An Experiential Approach to Behavior Change.* New York: Guilford Press.

Helgeson, V. S., and B. H. Gottlieb. 2000. Support groups. In *Social support measurement and intervention: A guide for health and social scientists,* ed. S. Cohen, L. G. Underwood, and B. H. Gottlieb. New York: Oxford University Press.

Horgen, K. B., and K. D. Brownell. 2002. Confronting the toxic environment: Environmental public health actions in a world crisis. In *Handbook of obesity treatment,* ed. T. A. Wadden and A. J. Stunkard. New York: Guilford Press.

International Center for Alcohol Policies (ICAP). 2007. www.icap.org/PolicyIssues/DrinkingGuidelines/StandardUnitsTable/tabid/253/Default.aspx.

Jakicic, J., R. R. Wing, and C. Winters. 1999. Effects of intermittent exercise and use of home exercise equipment on adherence, weight loss, and fitness in overweight women. *Journal of the American Medical Association* 282(16):1554–60.

Jeffrey, R. W., A. Drewnowski, L. H. Epstein, A. J. Stunkard, G. T. Wilson, and R. R. Wing. 2000. Long-term maintenance of weight loss: Current status. *Health Psychology* 19:5–16.

Johnson, C. 2002. Obesity, weight management, and self-esteem. In *Handbook of obesity treatment.* ed. T. A. Wadden and A. J. Stunkard. New York: Guilford Press.

Laliberte, M., M. Newton, R. McCabe, and J. S. Mills. 2007. Controlling your weight versus controlling your lifestyle: How beliefs about weight control affect risk for disordered eating, body dissatisfaction, and self-esteem. *Cognitive Therapy and Research* 31:853–69.

Lee, C. D., S. N. Blair, and A. S. Jackson. 1999. Cardiorespiratory fitness, body composition, and all-cause and cardiovascular disease mortality in men. *American Journal of Clinical Nutrition* 69:373–80.

Levy, A. S., and A. W. Heaton. 1993. Weight control practices in U.S. adults trying to lose weight. *Annals of Internal Medicine* 119(Suppl. 2):661–66.

Low, C. A., A. L. Stanton, and J. E. Bower. 2008. Effects of acceptance-oriented versus evaluative emotional processing on heart rate recovery and habituation. *Emotion* 8:419–24.

McGuire, M. X., R. R. Wing, M. L. Klem, and J. O. Hill. 1999. Behavioral strategies of individuals who have maintained long-term weight losses. *Obesity Research* 7:334–41.

Melanson, K., and J. Dwyer. 2002. Popular diets for treatment of overweight and obesity. In *Handbook of obesity treatment*, ed. T. A. Wadden and A. J. Stunkard. New York: Guilford Press.

Miller, W. R., and S. Rollnick. 2002. *Motivational Interviewing: Preparing People for Change.* New York: Guilford Press.

Mitchell, J. E., T. Cook Myers, L. Swan-Kremeier, and M. de Zwaan. 2006. The role of bariatric surgery in the obese patient with psychopathology. In *Obesity and mental disorders*, ed. S. L. McElroy, D. B. Allison, and G.A. Bray. New York: Taylor and Francis Group.

Mulheim, L.S., D. B. Allison, S. Heshka, and S. B. Heymsfield. 1998. Do unsuccessful dieters intentionally underreport food intake? *International Journal of Eating Disorders* 24:259–66.

Orzano, A. J., and J. G. Scott. 2004. Diagnosis and treatment of obesity in adults: An applied evidence-based review. *Journal of American Board Family Practice* 17:359–69.

Perri, M. G., R. M. Shapiro, W. W. Ludwig, C. T. Twentyman, and W. G. McAdoo. 1984. Maintenance strategies for the treatment of obesity: An evaluation of relapse prevention training and posttreatment contact by mail and telephone. *Journal of Consulting and Clinical Psychology* 52:404–13.

Prochaska, J. O., J. C. Norcross, and C. C. DiClemente. 1994. *Changing for Good: A Revolutionary Six-Stage Program for Overcoming Bad Habits and Moving Your Life Positively Forward.* New York: Avon.

Rosen, J. C., and T. F. Cash. 1995. Learning to have a better body image. *Weight Control Digest* 5:411–16.

Sarwer, D. B., J. K. Thompson, J. E. Mitchell, and J. P. Rubin. 2008. Psychological considerations of the bariatric surgery patient undergoing body contouring surgery. *Plastic and Reconstructive Surgery* 121:423e–34e.

Stathopoulou, G., M. B. Powers, A. C. Berry, J. A. J. Smits, and M. W. Otto. 2006. Exercise interventions for mental health: A quantitative and qualitative review. *Clinical Psychology: Science and Practice* 13:179–93.

Stotland, S., and D. C. Zuroff. 1990. A new measure of weight locus of control: The Dieting Beliefs Scale. *Journal of Personality Assessment* 54:191–203.

Stunkard, A., K. Allison, and J. Lundgren. 2008. Issues for DSM-V: Night eating syndrome. *American Journal of Psychiatry* 165:424.

Stunkard, A. J., J. R. Harris, N. L. Pederson, and G. E. McClearn. 1990. The body-mass index of twins who have been reared apart. *New England Journal of Medicine* 322:1483–87.

van Hout, G. C., F. A. Fortuin, A. J. Pelle, and G. L. van Heck. 2008. Psychosocial functioning, personality, and body image following vertical banded gastroplasty. *Obesity Surgery* 18:115–20.

Wadden, T. A., and R. I. Berkowitz. 2002. Very-low-calorie diets. In *Eating disorders and obesity: A comprehensive handbook,* 2nd ed., ed. C. G. Fairburn and K. D. Brownell. New York: Guilford Press.

Wadden, T. A., D. B. Sarwer, M. E. Arnold, D. Gruen, and P. M. O'Neil. 2000. Psychosocial status of severely obese patients before and after bariatric surgery. *Problems in General Surgery* 17:13–22.

Wadden, T. A., and A. J. Stunkard. 1985. Social and psychological consequences of obesity. *Annals of Internal Medicine* 103:1062–67.

Warburton, D. E., C. W. Nicol, and S. S. Bredin. 2006. Health benefits of physical activity: The evidence. *Canadian Medical Association Journal* 174:801–9.

Wilson, G. T., and K. D. Brownell. 2000. Behavioral treatment for obesity. In *Eating disorders and obesity: A comprehensive handbook,* 2nd ed., ed. C. G. Fairburn and K. D. Brownell. New York: Guilford Press.

Wing, R. R., and J. O. Hill. 2001. Successful weight loss maintenance. *Annual Review of Nutrition* 21:323–41.

World Health Organization. 1998. *Obesity: Preventing and Managing the Global Epidemic* (Publication No. WHO/NUT/NCD/98.1). Geneva: World Health Organization.

Yermilov, I, M. L. McGory, P. W. Shekelle, C. Y. Ko, and M. A. Maggard. 2009. Appropriateness criteria for bariatric surgery: Beyond the NIH guidelines. *Obesity,* 17:1521-7. Epub

Yusuf, S., S. Hawken, S. Ounpuu, L. Bautista, M. G. Franzosi, P. Commerford, C. C. Lang, Z. Rumboldt, C. L. Lisheng, S. Tanomsup, P. Wangai Jr., F. Razak, A. M. Sharma, and S. S. Anand; INTERHEART Study Investigators. 2005. Obesity and the risk of myocardial infarction in 27,000 participants from 52 countries: A case-control study. *Lancet* 366(9497):1640–49.

Michele Laliberte, Ph.D., is a clinical psychologist and director of the outpatient adult eating disorders program at St. Joseph's Healthcare in Hamilton, ON, Canada. She is also assistant professor in the department of psychiatry and neurosciences at McMaster University. She has trained numerous health care professionals in both individual and group cognitive behavioral therapy (CBT) treatment for eating disorders. She has published articles about the role of weight control beliefs and family factors that predict disturbed eating, and has presented at international conferences on eating disorders.

Randi E. McCabe, Ph.D., is psychologist-in-chief and director of the anxiety treatment and research center at St. Joseph's Healthcare in Hamilton, ON, Canada. She is also associate professor in the department of psychiatry and behavioral neurosciences at McMaster University. Her research has focused on anxiety, eating disorders, and cognitive behavioral therapy. She has published numerous articles and coauthored four books, including the *Overcoming Bulimia Workbook*.

Valerie Taylor, MD, Ph.D., is assistant professor in psychiatry and behavioral neurosciences at McMaster University in Hamilton, ON, Canada. At St. Joseph's Healthcare in Hamilton, she is director of the mood disorders somatic health program and heads the psychiatric team affiliated with the bariatric surgery program. Taylor's research focuses on the interrelations of addiction, obesity, and mental health. She has received numerous research grants and academic awards and has published extensively on the areas of obesity and physical health outcomes in patients with mental illness.

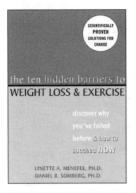
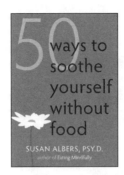
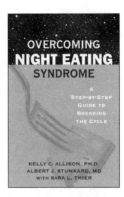
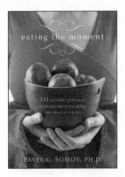
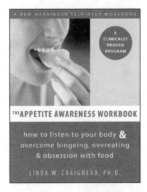
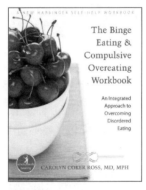